Stephen K. Wickman, Sr.

OVERCOMING YOUR
BROKEN HEART

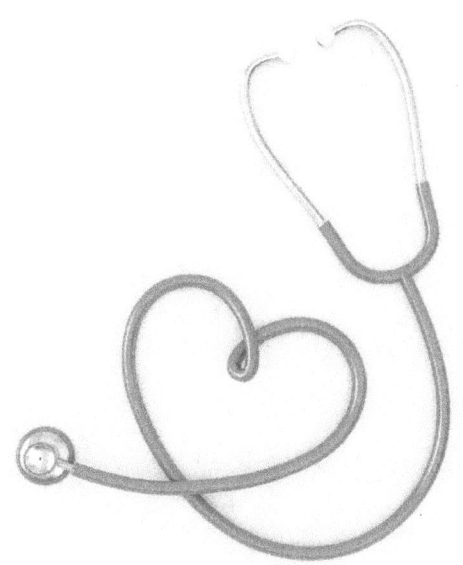

One Man's Incredible Journey:
Heart Disease:
What if It Happens to You?

Overcoming Your Broken Heart...

One Man's Incredible Journey:
Heart Disease:
What if it Happens to You?

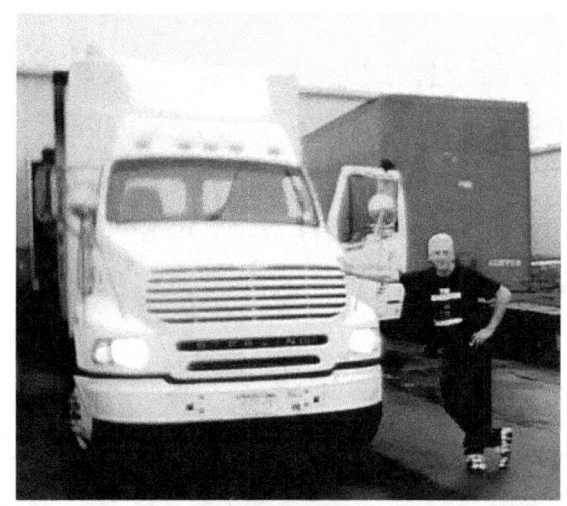

Ride Along As I Share My Journey
With You

By Stephen K. Wickman, Sr.

Overcoming Your Broken Heart:
One Man's Incredible Journey:
Heart Disease: What if it Happens to You?

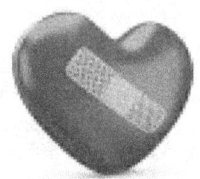

© 2012 Stephen K. Wickman, Sr.

No part of this book may be reproduced, stored in a retrieval system, or transmitted by any means without the written permission of the author.

First published: April 2012.
All rights reserved.

Printed in the United States of America

ISBN 9-78-1-105-33771-4

Dedication

This book is dedicated to the cardiac care team at the Rochester General Hospital in Rochester, NY, my care team in the Cardio Rehabilitation Department of the Newark Wayne Community Hospital (NWCH) in Newark, NY and to my care team in the Speech Pathology Department at NWCH. Thank you for all that you have done in helping me in my wellness journey. Words cannot express my deep gratitude to you all.

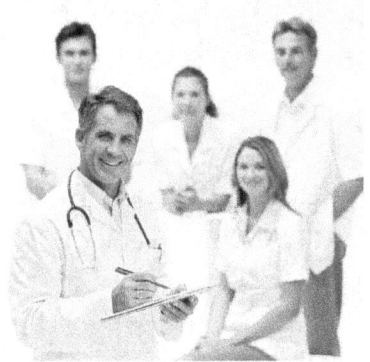

Thanks,
Steve

Thanks

A special thank you to Dr. Cynthia Huling Hummel for her help, support and guidance in preparing this manuscript.

Thanks to Jay Palmer for his assistance in helping to restore some photos for this book.

Thanks to Dorothy Mauser, Bruno K. Krause, Kenneth Warner, Crystal Roder, and Kathy Bement for providing me with valuable feedback on my manuscript.

Thanks to my family, friends and fellow patients for their support and encouragement.

Thanks to my fellow Toastmasters for encouraging me to share my journey to wellness.

THANK YOU!!!

 Thanks to a GREAT medical team: for their care, support, and assistance.

Dr. Krishna V. Persaud, MD
Internal Medicine

John F. Centonze, MD Otolaryngologist

Anita Prasad, C.N.P Dermatology & Family Practice

Cheryl Gilbert, RN and Sr. Clinician III

Kathy Blazey, RN and BSN

Geriann Jackson, M.S., CCC-SLP

Carol Henn-Staino, Au. D CC-A

Lawrence E. Gage, MD FACC

David C. Cheeran, MD Thoracic and Cardiac Surgery

Meet The Author: Steve Wickman

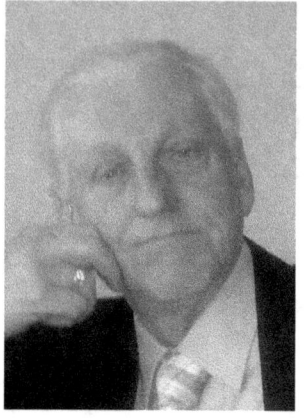

My name is Steve Wickman Sr. I am not a doctor or a nurse and I do not work in the health field. However, three years ago in 2008, I had triple bypass surgery and I want to tell you my story.

For a number of years before my by-pass surgery, I was a volunteer fire fighter and an emergency medical technician (EMT) in the county. Periodically I also rode with Advanced Life Support (A.L.S.) Unit Medic 88. I have performed cardiopulmonary resuscitation (CPR) in emergency situations. So I had seen heart related issues first hand.

FAMILY HISTORY OF CARDIAC PROBLEMS

Also for years, there have been cardiac problems in my own family. My older brothers both had heart issues. My son Stephen had heart related problems. When he was just one month old, he had open heart surgery to repair a hole in his heart and to correct a problem with reversed arteries. Six weeks later, he had another surgery to correct more problems. When he was three years old, he had another surgery. Stephen is 35 years old now, on his 5th pacemaker, and doing well. A HUGE thank you to Dr. Manning and the wonderful team at Strong Memorial Hospital in Rochester, NY.

Although I have been around heart problems much of my life, I never thought that a heart related problem awaited me: but here we are. This book is a look through one patient's eyes from the onset of my cardiac problems, my surgery, and my recovery in rehabilitation.

A PATIENT'S PERSPECTIVE

This book is not intended to tell you what to do with your condition or how to deal with your condition. You should always follow the advice of your caregiver. However this book is intended to let you see a cardiac incident from a patient's perspective. Perhaps it will give you a chuckle, or maybe bring a tear to your eye. Hopefully you will see that you are not alone. Many people have cardiac problems similar to mine and to yours. Perhaps reading this book will help you on your journey to wellness.

I hope you enjoy it!

Steve

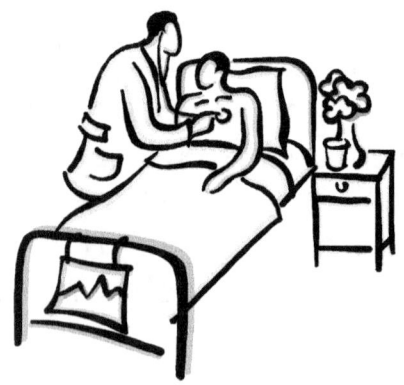

FORWARD

Although this book is my own story in my own words, I hope that the point being made will help all who are undergoing any type of illness, injury, or disease such as cancer, Alzheimer's, diabetes, muscular dystrophy, cardiovascular, and Hodgkin's, to name a few.

All injuries and diseases are different in nature as are the recommended treatments that are advised for that particular disorder. However, the effect on the patient and the families are very much the same.

I think that when we are confronted with a health issue, we all become scared and
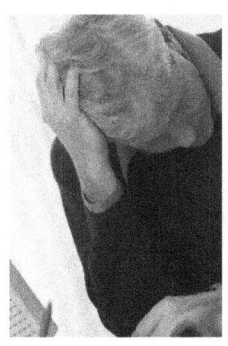
nervous, and have many questions that we seek answers to. We have many mixed emotions and uncertainties. We are not sure of why this has happened or what the outcome may be.

NEVER QUITE PREPARED

Let's face it when we go to the doctor for an annual check-up or because we have a problem that has surfaced, we hope for the best and are extremely relieved when we find out that what we have is very treatable and our outlook is good. On the other hand, we are never quite prepared for the news that we have a serious or devastating illness that we may not survive. And admit it or not, that thought is likely in the back of your mind. It was in mine. Being told all is good is far better than getting the news that this is very, very serious and suddenly finding yourself in the fight of your life for your life.

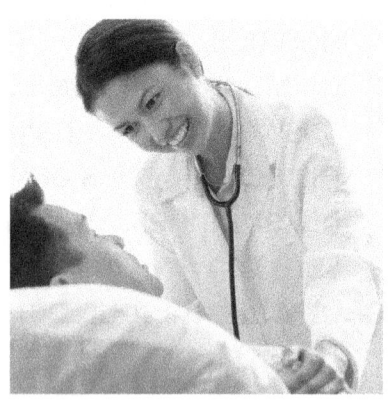

TAKE CARE OF YOURSELF NOW

Doing all that you can now to take care of yourself and lessen the chance of a serious problem down the road is what this book is about. Regardless of your condition or illness, we have the same goal and that is to get better. We have questions that we want answered. We all have things that we would still like to do. We all share the mixed emotions and feelings that arise and we all have treatments and procedures that we must face.

Being scared and frustrated, angry and hurt, having pain and discomfort, not knowing what lies ahead in the days or weeks to come are some of the many feelings and thoughts that we all face. Regardless of our own diagnosis, we are all receiving some kind of treatment and we all want a favorable outcome.

DO WHAT YOU CAN NOW

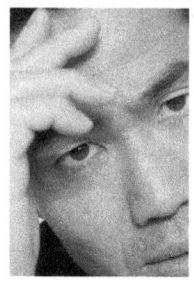 Look at your family history. Do all that you can to live a healthier lifestyle. Try and do all that you can do now to lessen the chance of illness down the road. Take better care of yourself now while you can and if you are experiencing any health issues, seek treatment immediately. Do not wait! Call your health care provider and should you not have one, seek one out! If you are hesitant, I hope that what I have written will help convince you to seek medical advice and care. If you are undergoing any kind of treatment, I hope while you are reading this, that you will find that you are not alone. I also am like you with thousands of others just like us, doing all that we can with the help of many wonderful professionals to live a healthier, longer, fruitfully happy life.

LISTEN TO YOUR BODY

We all need to listen to our bodies and address what we hear. We need to have regular checkups. Most of all, we need to seek medical help as soon as we realize that something is wrong. No one wants to get hurt. No one wants to get sick, and certainly no one wants to die needlessly. So let's do all that we can now. It is never too late to stay healthy, get better, recover nicely, and live each day to its fullest.

YOUR ATTITUDE MATTERS

Some of us will not get sick. Some of us will recover nicely. Some of us will succumb to our illness, but we all can give thanks for each day and always keep the hope alive for a better tomorrow. Share your dreams and hopes and make the most out of each and every day that you and I have left. Your personal outlook and determination will carry you a long way on your journey to wellness. Regardless of the outcome make each second count.   Be well and the very best of luck to you! *Steve*

MY WISH FOR YOU

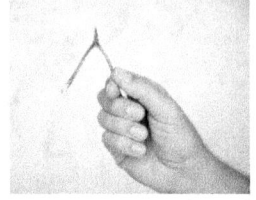 If you are scheduled for any kind of cardiac procedure or have had corrective measures taken, I hope that this book will help you better understand what to expect and help you on your way to a better tomorrow.

It is a true life look through one patient's eyes on my experience from the onset of my cardio problems to the ongoing treatments that I still receive today. We will look at things from the patient's true experience and perspective and how I have coped with the issues at hand.

MY STORY

This book is not in any way meant to give medical advice or tell anyone how to feel. IT IS ONLY MEANT TO SHARE MY STORY WITH YOU in the hopes you will strive to take better care of yourself, seek medical support, and realize that you are not alone.

I live in upstate New York. I was born in 1952 and have worked since I was in my teens as a farm hand, laborer, truck driver, sales person, and musician, just to name a few. At age 56, I had a heart attack and five months later, I had triple bypass surgery. As I write this, it is now three years later and at age 59, I still go to cardio rehabilitation 3-4 times weekly.

This is my story of the ups and downs that I have experienced along the way. I hope you find it comforting and an enjoyable reading experience. Now sit back and let me share my story with you. But first I want to say a word to those of you who might be reading and haven't experienced a cardiac episode and are wondering if this book is for you. Well, keep reading!

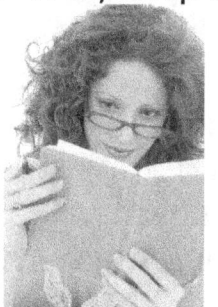

FOR YOU HEALTHY READERS

First of all, congratulations! For those of you who are healthy and have no signs or symptoms of cardiovascular disease or heart ailments, that's wonderful. Let's do all we can to ensure that you stay this way. I hope that you continue to have a long and happy healthy life. Perhaps in reading this book, you will see how sometimes in the course of our life, changes happen. Illness can slowly begin and sneak up on us before we know it.

One day I was 5 years old and starting school. Then in a blink of an eye, I was 12 years old and could not wait to be a teenager. Then suddenly, I was 15 looking towards 16 and being able to drive. My teenage years led to my 20's getting married and starting a family. Then came 35, middle age and time really started flying by then. Wow, what a glorious time. One day I turned Nifty Fifty. I was still feeling good and looking good (for my age) and still enjoying life and not looking back. Then at age 56, cardiovascular disease came to visit and stayed.

THE POINT I AM MAKING

The point I am making is this: Do all that you can do regardless of your age to address your health issues. Do all that you can do now to prevent the illness and diseases that seem to sneak up on us as we grow older. Continue to seek advice as you continue on your life's journey about how to maintain good health. As you read along you may notice some mistakes that <u>I made</u> along the way, that you may be able to avoid, hopefully saving you some issues of your own, down the road of life.

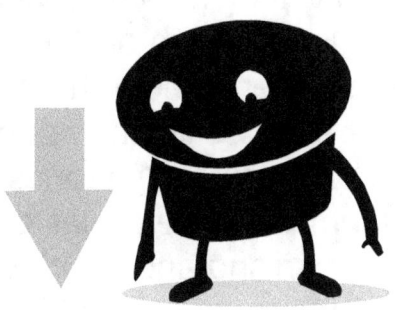

THIS CAN HELP YOU TO UNDERSTAND WHAT IT'S LIKE TO BE A CARDIAC PATIENT

As you read even now, knowing that you are fit and healthy and feeling just fine, you may see in my story, a similarity- perhaps with a loved one or friend that you know. Having an understanding of what can happen and what someone else is or has been dealing with, will give you a little insight into that person and the difficulties that people face when dealing with cardiac disease and personal health problems. I have found that I am a little more patient with people, who seem to be struggling with one problem or another. I often offer to help those who appear tired or sickly. I listen with more interest to an older person's stories and words of wisdom. You see, I was once just as you are now: strong and running. I was too busy living life to pay attention to what my lifestyle was slowly doing to my body.

FUNNY ISN'T IT?

Now here I am, a seasoned older fellow, sharing my adventures and stories with all who would listen. Funny isn't it? How when we are young and we think we know it all, when we really know nothing at all. Then as we grow older, we are too busy to appreciate what we have learned along the way. As we age, we often try so hard to roll back the clock and slow time down a bit and share our thoughts and wisdom with others, as so many did with us in our youth. Think about it. How many times did you listen to a story or were shown how to do something , sometimes over and over again, when you would much rather have made a trip to the dentist to have a tooth pulled or dig a ditch with a spoon.

IF I COULD DO IT OVER AGAIN

I would give anything to listen to one of the many stories of my youth just one more time right now. And I sure wish that I had taken the time to listen with a better understanding then, when I had the opportunity. I hope you will be encouraged to stay healthy and try to understand those of us who at this moment are not as fortunate as you are. So go ahead and enjoy life and all the wonderful bounties that it offers, but do so in a healthy way. It is never too late to start a better tomorrow and always the right time to learn and continue healthy habits that may increase your longevity. Good luck!

Steve

THE SAGA BEGINS...

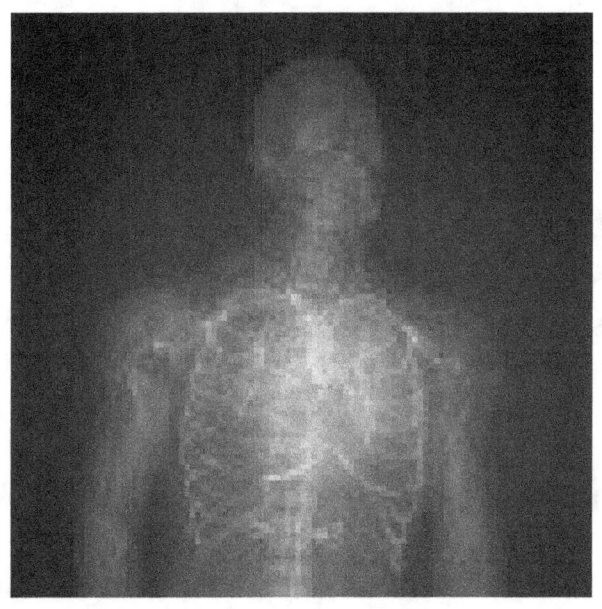

Or I had NO Idea what I was in for...

THE SAGA BEGINS:

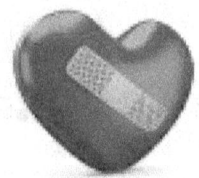

TUESDAY MORNING

"You better come over and look at this." I watched the doctor call two of his team members over to look at the screen. I wondered what was happening.   They all turned to me and one said, "Mr. Wickman, you have three total blockages and you need to go into surgery right now."

One of the doctors said, "I am going to give you some meds now to relax you." And after a shot, I was on the table being rushed down the hall to the operating room. I was watching the lights overhead fly by and thinking it looked like something out of a movie, except this time I was the star. Instead of watching the movie, though, I was in it; so much for a routine test.

MORE THAN A SMALL BLOCKAGE

I thought I had a small blockage of about 38%. I had a barrage of tests and was seeing my primary care physician and a cardiologist. I was taking meds, but wasn't feeling much better. I was scheduled for an angioplasty. This is where a camera is inserted into the artery near the groin to take a look inside your arteries, to find out what is going on. I kept thinking, "I should be feeling better," but I wasn't. Well now I knew why: I had three arteries that were blocked 98-99%. I've heard that doctors will sometimes call this condition the "widow maker" for obvious reasons. They rushed me to surgery.

BACKING UP A BIT

Perhaps I should back up a bit. All the signs of a heart problem were there, but I didn't heed them and I didn't take them seriously. I don't really know when my cardiac problems started, but at age 56, something was definitely wrong. What was puzzling was that I had always been active and in good physical shape (or so I THOUGHT).

Okay, I smoked. I ate "kind of right", and felt pretty good over-all. I knew that my blood pressure was high, so I exercised and tried to do everything myself. I was never really a "go to the doctor" kind of guy. I had heartburn all the time and ate Rolaids like m&m's. (This isn't an endorsement, just my preference!)

THE SUMMER OF MY HEART ATTACKS

It was summer and I was sweating a lot. I had a little tightness in my chest from time to time and gradually, it seemed to me to be getting worse. I was always on edge and anxious. Everyone said I was wound too tight and that I needed to chill. But with work and home, that was just everyday life to me. One day I was not feeling well at all. Everything was going wrong and while I was working on my lawnmower, I hit my hand. As if that didn't hurt enough, it was nothing compared to the pain that I felt in my chest. Thank God I already was bent over. Holy cow! The pain lasted about 10-15 seconds, but it felt like forever. Finally, it stopped and I got sick to my stomach. I threw up for 3 to 5 minutes, then it was over and I felt okay. I blamed it on the heat that day and what I had eaten for lunch. I rested a minute or so and went back to work. All was well, that is, until Monday.

THE 900 POUND GORILLA

On Monday I went to work. I work in sales. I was walking from one office into another when suddenly it felt like a 900lb gorilla hit me in the chest. The pain put me on the floor. I got up and asked our customer service rep who happened to be nearby what had happened. She said, "You just dropped, shook your head, then stood up."

IN RETROSPECT

She wanted to call an ambulance, but by then, I felt fine and told her, no. I already had a doctor's appointment scheduled for that afternoon, so I called my doctor and went right over to his office. It was a stupid move on my part. I should have gone by ambulance to the hospital, but being stubborn, I drove myself. I realize now, that I should have called for an ambulance, and I also should have called 9-1-1 the Saturday before, when I had the excruciating chest pain.   Like many, I denied that anything was wrong and found excuses for my chest pain instead.

THE MOMENT OF TRUTH

At the doctor's office, my EKG showed that I did indeed have something happen. My blood pressure and pulse were high, but by then, I was feeling okay. So after being checked over, I was sent to the hospital for more testing and met with a cardiologist.   I had a barrage of tests and then a stress test. I thought that I aced the stress test. True, I had a little tightness in my chest, but no pain and that's when the 38% blockage showed up, but nothing else at the time. So with new meds in hand and a new diet, I headed home.

A WALKING TIME BOMB

For four months, I did what I was told but still kept getting tightness in my chest. It

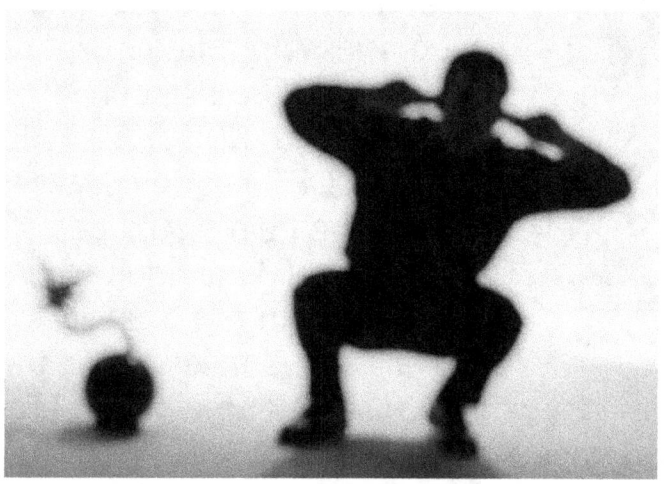

was coming more often and with little or no exercising. The tightness and pain got so bad that I couldn't walk more than 30-50 feet without having to stop to let the tightness subside and still I denied that anything was wrong.

UNABLE TO USE A PUSH BROOM

I couldn't even use a push broom to clean my shop. Anything I did with my arms 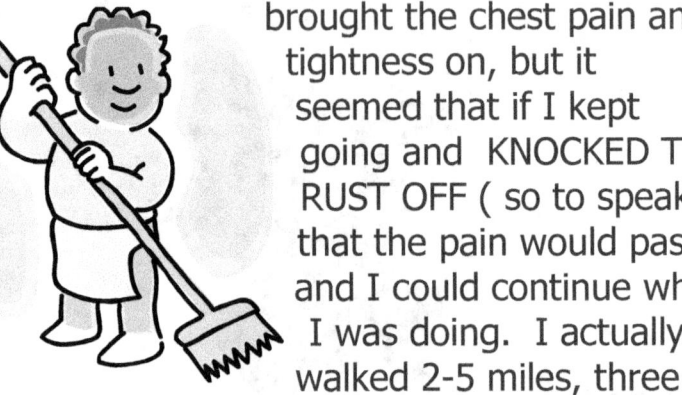 brought the chest pain and tightness on, but it seemed that if I kept going and KNOCKED THE RUST OFF (so to speak), that the pain would pass and I could continue what I was doing. I actually walked 2-5 miles, three to four times a week. Once I got moving, it all seemed good. I assumed that I just needed more time for my body to adjust to the meds. Little did I know, I was a walking time bomb waiting to explode. I wasn't paying attention to "The Signs."

KNOW THE SIGNS

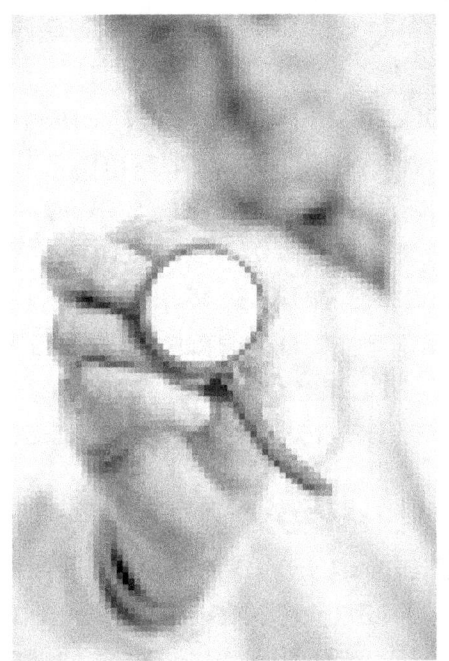

HEART ATTACKS: KNOW THE SIGNS!

If you are like me, perhaps you think that all heart attacks are sudden and intense — like the kind that you see in the movies where the man clutches his chest and falls to the ground dead as a door nail. Hey everyone in the theater knows what is happening. But most heart attacks, I'm told, start slowly, with a mild pain or discomfort. Sometimes people aren't even sure what's wrong and they wait too long before getting help. This is what I've learned about possible warning signs that you may be having a heart attack.

CHEST DISCOMFORT.

I had tightness in my chest, but I never thought my heart was trying to tell me something. If you have pain or discomfort in the center of the chest, get help immediately. I felt at times like an elephant was sitting on my chest. I also experienced heartburn all the time. So if you are feeling pressure, in your chest, have it checked out pronto.

PAIN OR DISCOMFORT IN OTHER AREAS OF THE UPPER BODY.

I've heard that the warning signs for heart attacks may include pain or discomfort in one or both arms, in your back, neck, jaw or stomach. So again, don't wait! Seek medical advice.

SHORTNESS OF BREATH.

If you are having trouble breathing i.e. shortness of breath, with or without chest pain, get it checked out. It could be a warning sign of a cardiac problem or other serious illness.

OTHER SIGNS.

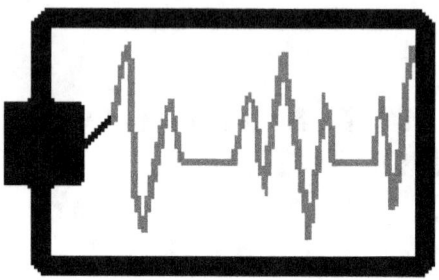

Believe it or not, other symptoms of a cardiac problem might be..

♥ breaking out in a cold sweat

♥ nausea

♥lightheadedness

♥ a constant feeling of indigestion.

Again, don't wait or hesitate to get medical advice. It may be more than the flu!

WOMEN'S SYMPTOMS

I have read that a woman's most common heart attack symptoms are a dull ache in the

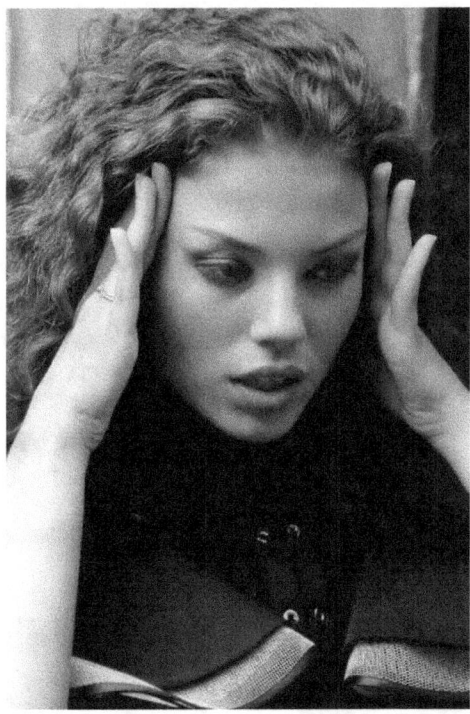

back between the shoulder blades, increasing fatigue, and **chest pain or discomfort**. But I have also been told that women are more likely than men to experience some of the other common symptoms. These include: **shortness of breath, Nausea/vomiting, and back or jaw pain**.

LEARN THE SIGNS

Learn the signs and remember this: Even if

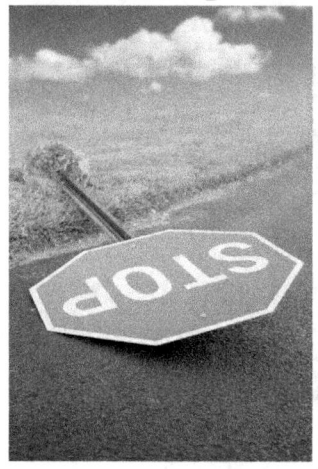

you're not sure it's a heart attack, please have it checked out. Tell a doctor about your symptoms. Sometimes, people are afraid to seek medical help unless they feel it is a true medical emergency. Sometimes people make the excuse that they don't have the time to be checked out. Sometimes they are afraid that it might not be a heart problem and that they would be embarrassed. Don't make excuses. Get help now. **Remember call 9-1-1.**

CALLING 9-1-1

Calling 911 is almost always the fastest way to get lifesaving treatment. I worked as an EMT for many years, and I can tell you this, emergency medical services (EMS) staff can start treatment when they arrive. They are trained and equipped to revive someone who is in cardiac arrest or having any medical emergency.

DON'T TAKE A CHANCE

Don't take a chance. Call 911. You might think, I'll just have my wife (or husband) drive me to the hospital. But what if you stop breathing? What would your loved one do? Please don't put yourself or your loved one in this position.

NO DRIVING ALLOWED

Also, please don't even think about driving yourself to the hospital. Suppose you pass out? Suppose you hit another vehicle or a person? Do NOT I repeat, do NOT drive yourself to the hospital. Call 911. Thank you!

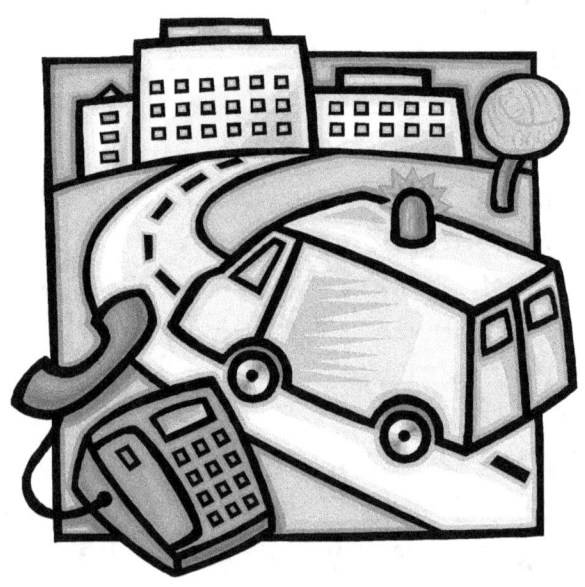

WHAT WERE MY SIGNS AND SYMPTOMS?

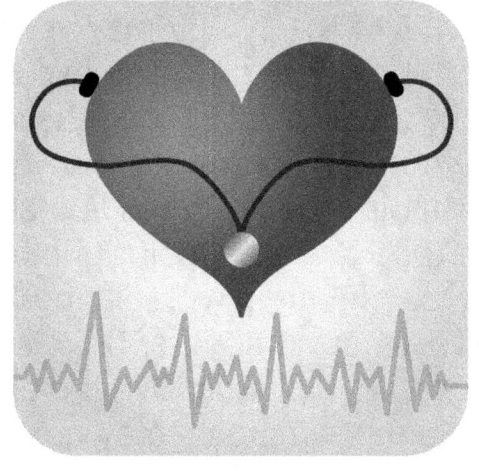

PAIN

NAUSEA

VOMITING

TIGHTNESS IN CHEST

SHORTNESS OF BREATH

TIREDNESS

UNABLE TO SLEEP WELL

TENSE AND ANXIOUS

MAKING EXCUSES

Yes, I had ALL of the symptoms I've listed at one time or another and I made excuses for every one of them. Please heed the signs. You know your body better than anyone. Listen to what it is trying to tell you and call your doctor or 911. As a point of interest, I didn't have pain in my jaw, radiating pain in my arm or back or numbness, but I was still in big trouble. REMEMBER: We are all different. So my symptoms may not be yours. I'm not a doctor, I'm just sharing my experiences. You need to see YOUR health care provider who can run diagnostics. Please don't wait to seek help.

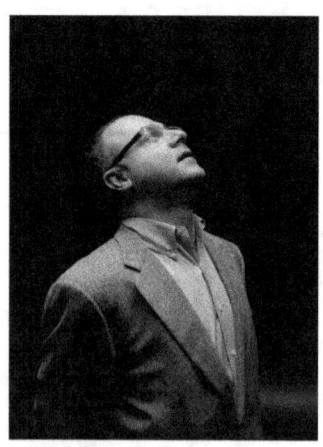

MY SAGA CONTINUES:

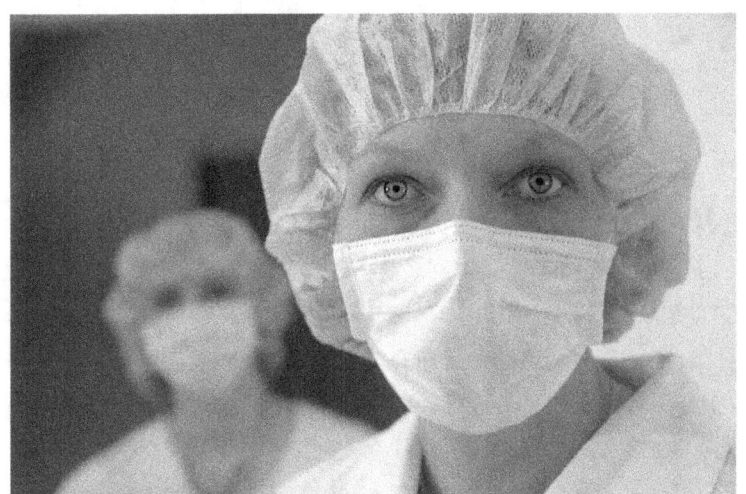

Emergency Surgery,
A Near Death Experience,
& A Slow Recovery

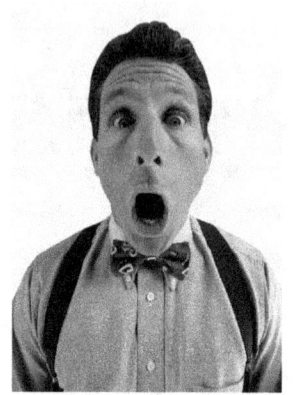

SHOCKING NEWS

So back to my story. I had gone to get some tests. I thought I might be having an angioplasty and was pretty sure that I would be home that night (or certainly by the next day), basically as "good as new." So I was not prepared when the doctors told me that I was in major trouble and would be heading to surgery right then and there. It was like a bad dream. I was numb and cold. I was on a gurney being prepped and we were racing down the hall. It was like something you see on the TV.

PRE-OP (OR FIVE MINUTES OF ANGER AND FRUSTRATION)

When we arrived at the operating room, we stopped outside the door so I could quickly see my family, and meet my surgeon and my cardio team. It allowed me to chat a few minutes before we got started. I was pretty sedated but I was also angry. I thought, "How could this be happening to me now when I thought I was on the road to recovery months earlier? I was heading into surgery confused, scared and angry. I had my son, Stephen call a pastor. He handed me the phone and I asked for prayers.

AN ANGRY MOMENT

I was angry and after reading my cardiologist the riot act, I proceeded to tell the surgeon that if he could not care for me, as he would his own mother or father, sister or brother, son or daughter, dog or cat- not to even pick up the knife. I did not want him or anyone touching me unless they truly cared about me.

IN GOOD HANDS

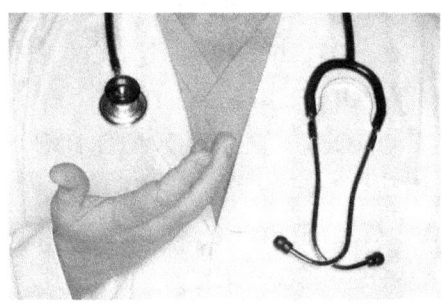 It got pretty quiet for a minute. My cardiologist explained to me that widow makers sometimes do not show up in tests. He assured me that everyone there cared about me and my well-being. He reminded me that I was lucky that my blockages were found and that I didn't drop dead long before then. My cardiologist told me that I had The BEST surgeon and team; that I was in one of the TOP ranked heart hospitals in the world and they would do everything in their power to assure a good outcome. Not feeling much better, I said goodbye to all and away we went.

AN EMERGENCY PROCEDURE

I remember thinking to myself, "Oh man! I hope I didn't tick them off! But oh well, it's too late now here we go." As for the operation, I really don't remember anything. It was much later when I learned the details of the event: that I had a triple bypass surgery and it took hours and hours. The surgeon and his team took veins from my left leg and from my chest which they used in the grafting process around my blockages.

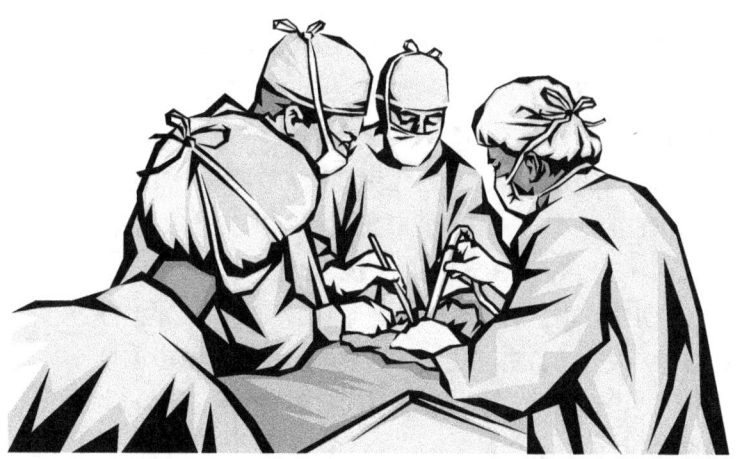

THE ANGEL

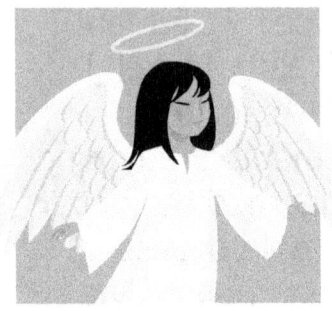 I was spinning out of control in total darkness. It was kind of like laying flat on your back, on a merry-go- round, spinning faster and faster- clockwise and it seemed to go lower and lower. I was in total darkness, spinning faster and asking God to take me and make it stop. I didn't know if I was heading up or heading down, but I knew that I couldn't take any more. Then I saw a dim light and a hand coming to me out of the darkness, but I could not grab it. I was spinning too fast. Gradually, the spinning slowed and I finally could grasp the hand. I knew then that I was coming back and the hand of the angel held on to my hand and a soft beautiful voice told me, "I won't let you go." And I could barely make out the words, but I finally felt calm and hope and love. And whatever would be would be, but it would be all right. That much I knew.

INTENSIVE CARE

I slowly opened my eyes. It was 5:20 by the clock on the wall. I could not move or talk. Two men were at the foot of the bed and a woman was at my head, though I could not see her, I felt her presence. I was in Intensive Care in guarded condition and they were slowly waking me up. I was uncomfortable and in pain but it was NOT unbearable. I had no idea where I was, what had happened, and what was going to happen. I was totally confused and heavily medicated.

WHAT DAY IS IT?

I was told I had quite a rough time, but that things were looking up and they would be slowly waking me up. I thought that my operation must have gone pretty well. I came in at 7 am for the angioplasty, went to surgery shortly thereafter and it was only 5:20 that night. Then one of the men said, "Do you know what day it is???"

NEEDING TO PEE

I had lost a day and a half. Wow. I went back to sleep. Sometime later, I awoke again and man did I have to pee. I could not talk or move but finally one of the men said, "Steve? What's wrong? Do you have to pee?"

My eyes were about blowing out of my head, so I guess they got the message that I really had to pee and bad! The nurse laughed and said, "Go ahead. You have a catheter and you can go any time." As I filled the bag, he turned to the other nurse and said. "I have never seen anyone hold it with a cath in before. I think he's going to be okay."

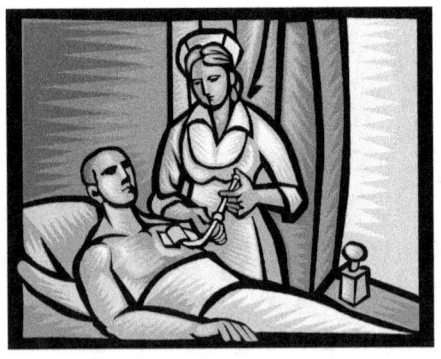

TUBES EVERYWHERE

I had tubes everywhere: in my neck, down my throat, up my nose and probably places I still don't know about, but they all had a purpose and I was alive. As I became more alert, I was told that if everything went okay that I would be weaned off some of this stuff and maybe, if I was lucky, be moved to a room later that night. It had become a very long day. The two guys were surgical intensive care nurses as was the lady by my head whom I never saw. I also was told that they constantly watched over me for many hours. I was their patient and they would not and did not want to leave me until I was stable. I guess I made a impression on them. I sure showed them that I could hold my water.

I also found out that after my surgery my heart stopped two times and I was paddled more than once to bring me back and they were not about to lose me. Hmmm. That would explain the red marks on my chest and sides that I would question later.

THANK YOU TO MY TEAM

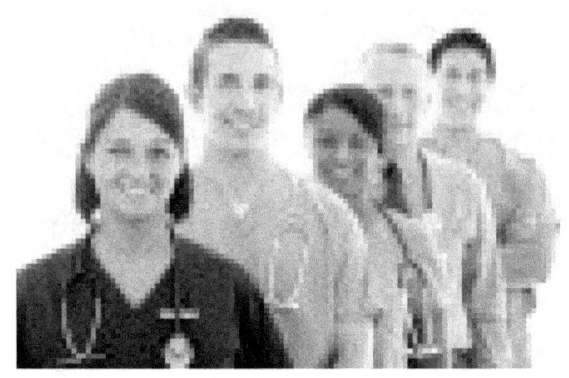

THANK YOU ALL FOR THE WONDERFUL CARE THAT YOU GAVE TO ME AND EVERYONE ELSE WHOM YOU HAVE HAD AS A PATIENT. YOU ARE A CREDIT TO YOUR PROFESSION AND I WILL ALWAYS BE INDEBTED TO YOU, MY BELOVED CAREGIVERS.

VISITORS

I could have a few visitors for a few brief moments. I really don't remember too much. I couldn't talk, but I could blink. People came in a blur, but it was nice. Then came nighttime again. I was told that there was quite a commotion that occurred shortly thereafter. You see, an IV stand is not supposed to be a coat rack- not even an empty one like the one that was by my bed. One of my visitors (no, it was not my SISTER) hung her coat on it, causing it to fall over on my bed, sending me into orbit. IT WAS AN ACCIDENT. Well I got sedated and sent back to sleep and everyone got tossed out on their fannies. I would not be able to have any visitors now until I was moved upstairs. But I must say the second round of sleep was better than the first. I was out like a light.

WAKING UP

Waking up again and slowly getting some of my senses back, over a period of days, I was cautiously weaned off the ventilator. Finally they removed the tube out of my neck- that one was a pain in the neck- literally, and I got my first wet sponge across my lips. It was like Christmas! It felt so good! Then came a glass of ice a few hours later. That was soooooo gooooood. I was finally awake, though groggy, and was able to be filled in on what had happened, what was done, and where I would be heading next. It was great to be alive again !!!

WEDNESDAY NIGHT

It was now Wednesday evening around 7:30pm. I had come in for my test on Tuesday at 7 am. The realization and enormity of all that had happened was starting to take place as I was being prepped to be moved upstairs to the cardio ward.

A NEW ROOM ON A NEW FLOOR

It was still Intensive Care but not as intense,

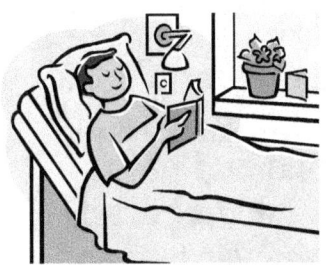 I guess. My two male nurses were still with me looking a little tired but happy for me. They filled me in on how to ease any pain by making sure that I asked for my pain medication before it ran out. They took me up to get settled, thanked me for being a good patient, and wished me well. I was almost sorry to see them go. They took good care of me.

SO GRATEFUL

As a note to readers: One month after my surgery, I went back to thank them and to meet the people who stayed by me for hours on end. I am so grateful and talking with them all was very emotional but so fulfilling. "Thank you" means a lot to everyone. Don't be afraid to say, "Thanks."

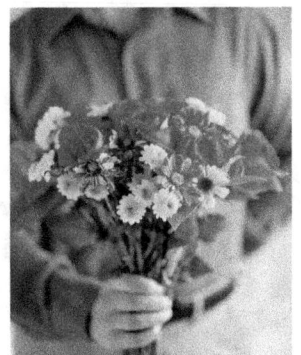

HELL WOULD FREEZE OVER FIRST

I was taken upstairs and placed in a room with another gentleman. At the time, neither one of us felt much like talking. I was settled in and given some juice to drink and a nurse came by to say that they would be getting me up later to stand and be weighed. ARE YOU KIDDING ME!? I politely told her that hell would freeze over first and that tomorrow I would do whatever they wanted but tonight, I just wanted my pain meds and sleep... and tomorrow, food and then and only then would I get up. Yes, I was miserable and probably kind of a jerk, but she smiled and said, "Let's see. Shall we?" Well guess what? I got my way.

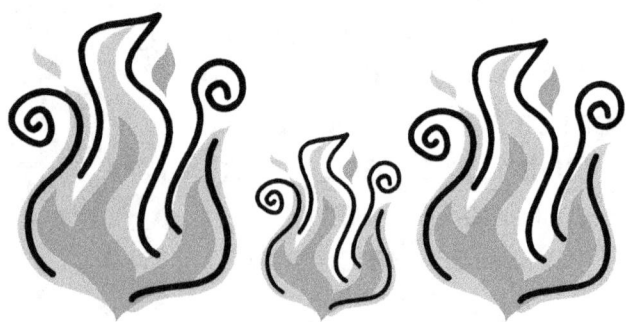

SPECIAL CARE

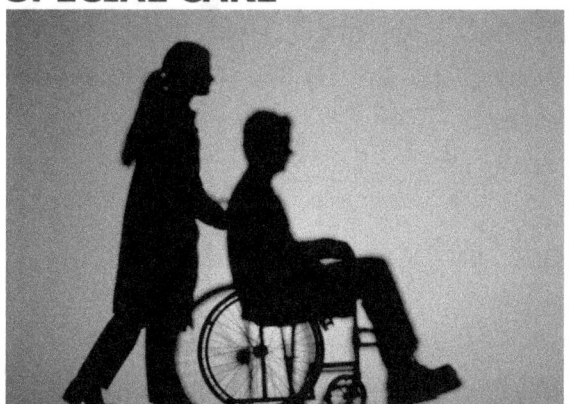

What a wonderful lady she was! I got meds every two hours. I got to sleep and when I couldn't sleep and seemed restless, she would come in, sit by my bed and hold my hand. She told me that everything would be okay and that her job was to take care of me and my job was to try and sleep and get better.

By the way did you ever notice that it seems they wake you up to see how you're doing and if you're sleeping okay when you are finally asleep? Interesting isn't it?

THURSDAY: STANDING AND WALKING

Okay, it's Thursday morning. I got pain meds. I know where I am and I'm going to get some food and COFFEE. Oh yeah! Let's rock.

"It's time to get up for a bit and stand," the nurse said.

I replied "Okie dokie. Let's go." I sat up ready to show them I was no sissy and that I was going to do it and get out of there and back to work in a day or two. I got ready to get up, looked down and saw my incision for the first time.

HOLY COW. Big Bird is yellow. A ghost is white. The Jolly Green Giant is green and I was BLUE. What the heck? Well, it was the cover over the incision and whatever they painted me with before surgery. It was a little shocking to see, but hey, it was a nice straight cut and actually made a nice definition in my chest. My pecs looked more defined. I tried to stand up and found out I had tubes, hoses, wires and stuff still all over me that required a team of engineers to assemble onto the IV pole before I could stand. Then with the nurse's help, I stood.

WEAK IN THE KNEES
A moment later, I realized I was not the man I thought I was. I was weak. I wobbled. I ached and like a little child getting up from a fall for the first time, I wondered if I could do it. Well guess what? With help, I did! Then I got to sit in the chair. And as the day went on, I walked with help and a walker. That day, I walked out the room and half way around the nurses' station. By that night, I walked all the way around the unit.   I was sore. I was tired, but I was determined and like cheerleaders, everyone coached me on while keeping a watchful eye.

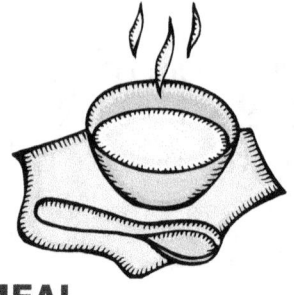

MY FIRST MEAL

By the end of that day, my mind wanted me to do more, while my body seemed to be holding me back. My nurses said something like I should try and get more rest and not to push it. "Boy, oh boy."

They delivered my first full hospital meal and the food was GREAT. Of course I didn't get the prime rib and crab legs I wanted, but the soup, mashed potatoes and jello were so good. I was tired and sore, but things were looking up.

HUGGIE PILLOWS: A MUST!

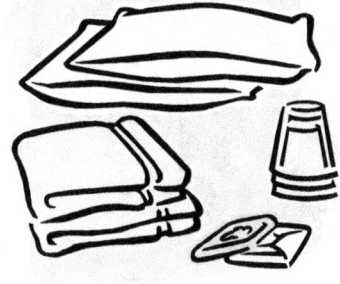 I also STRONGLY SUGGEST a Huggie pillow. You will be a little sore, but it sure helps to hug!!! A huggie pillow (also known as a cardiac pillow) is smaller than a regular pillow and it provides comfort and support to your chest area after your cardiac surgery.

USE YOUR PILLOW

It really helps to hold the pillow to your chest when you cough- and allows you to cough more efficiently, as you protect your healing incision and sutures. Some hospitals will personalize their cardiac pillows with a patient's name written on it or a drawing of a heart done with permanent magic marker. Some hospitals will let you take your cardiac pillow home. There are craft stores where you can buy heart shaped pillows if you'd like.

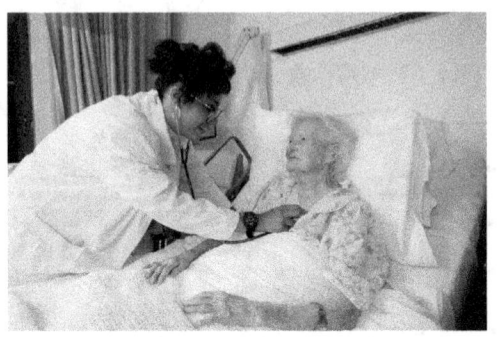

YOUR PAIN LEVEL

I slept pretty well, but make sure you ask for, get, and take your pain meds! They are given to you for a good reason: it hurts. Everyone's pain level is different. I'll admit it, I am a wussie. I do not like pain. But all in all, my pain was no where near what I envisioned it would be and if you listen to your doctor and nurses and do what they say, it's not that bad at all. Remember, your doctors and nurses are there to help you get stronger and better and sometimes they want you to do things you do not want to do. It is tough love, but they truly care. And the more you listen and harder you work at healing and getting better the easier it will be.

FRIDAY: MY FIRST SHOWER.

OKAY. I am up and walking with the walker. It's Friday morning and after my walk, I am told I can have a shower. It was probably a good thing. I can't smell anything, but I'm pretty sure that I am getting ripe. After all, they were wearing masks. I am helped into the shower along with my IV POLE. Yes, I am still wired up to stuff. My incision is covered but as I look down, I notice the tubes still sticking out of my mid-section. I guess they were some sort of drain tubes. Hmmm. With all the stuff going on, I never really noticed them before. Well okay. Nothing hurting, so here we go. Ahhh!! Man, did that shower feel good. With a fresh, new gown, my hair washed, and shaved, I feel like a new man.

THE TUBES COME OUT

After lunch, a nurse came in and said the surgeon would be in later that day. She asked if she could check my drain tubes. I said sure. She looked and said, "They look great. Take a deep breath for me. I want another peek."

I took a breath and what the heck was that? I just felt like someone pulled my stomach through my belly button. With tubes in her hand and a smile on her face, she said, "Now that wasn't bad, was it?"

"Gee whiz lady! You didn't tell me you were going to do that."

" I know," she said, "I wanted you to relax and let it be a surprise. It's much easier this way."

Well it sure was- for her. I think I understand why she did it that way and she really wasn't an EVIL WOMAN, though it seemed so at the time. She put a little gauze bandage over the three new little holes in my abdomen and left with a chuckle and a smile on her face. As she left, another nurse came in with my meds.

You can expect to be given a lot of pills, too many to figure out, but all are needed for your health and well-being. I would not kid you on this one.

NAPTIME

I have had a few visitors over the last three days and sadly, they seem to show up at nap time. I repeat this: Naptime is something you will look forward to in the weeks to come. It is a great part of your healing.

Rest is GOOD. So if you are tired, as much as you may want visitors, tell them you need the nap. They will understand.

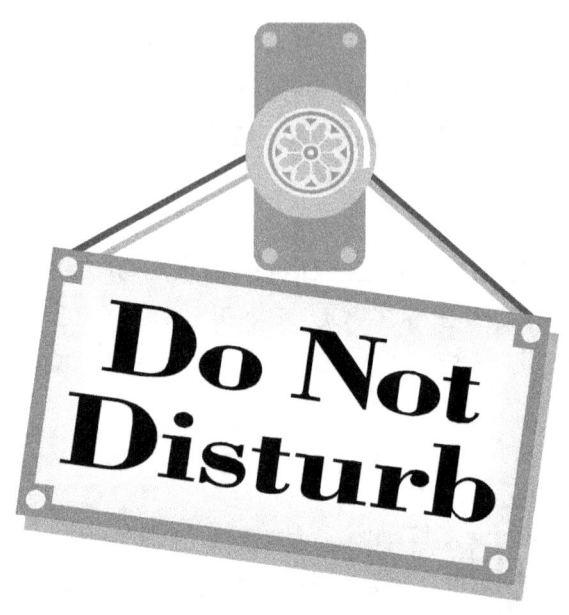

REST AND RECUPERATION GO HAND IN HAND

TAKE YOUR NAPS. YOUR BODY NEEDS THE SLEEP TO HEAL.

THE SUCKIE TOY (AKA THE SPIROMETER)

Almost as soon as I got to sleep, a doctor came in with what I call the "suckie toy." It's a device you have to use to improve and strengthen your lung function. Sorry! I forgot to mention this device earlier. You will meet this little rascal as soon as you get out of ICU. It will be your new friend. Don't be scared. It won't hurt you. It is all good. Your body has had quite a shock and it's all part of the healing process. The suckie toy doesn't HURT. Think of it as a challenge. I had races with the guy in the next bed to see who could raise the ball the farthest. We both won.

MEETING MY SURGEON.

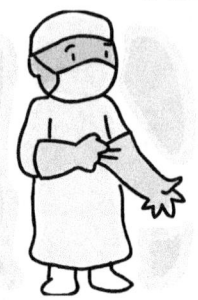 A group of nurses came in and unhooked almost all that was left on me and said, "We want you to get up, get weighed, and take a walk around the unit."

I said, "Okay." There was nothing on TV anyway at that time, so off I went. After the walk, I sat down in the chair. The nurses took my blood pressure, pulse and all the other stuff they check on and told me that the surgeon would be in to talk to me in a few moments.

" Okay. Now what's up ?" My mind was running wild when I heard a voice and saw a man dressed in green scrubs coming in the door. He introduced himself as my surgeon.

"Mr. Wickman?"

At first I didn't recognize him, but then I realized that he was the surgeon who saved my life.

"You look great after all that you've been through. I know you don't remember a lot, but you my friend had a triple bypass," which he then totally explained with charts and pictures that I really wasn't sure that I was ready to see yet.

He continued, "You also gave us a start when your heart decided to stop a couple times. That is why you have little paddle marks, those red marks on your sides.

You also had a little event in Surgical ICU when one of your visitors knocked an IV pole over onto your IV pole which then bounced off your respirator, which landed on you, and set off all sorts of alarms. It put you into orbit which then caused us to put you into a induced coma for a bit. We had to throw your guests out so we could take care of you. I think they understood the reason why. If not, tough.

Anyway, you did remarkably well and seem to be bouncing back nicely. I am very happy with the surgery and your recovery so far. In fact, you can go home Saturday afternoon or later today if you wish. It's up to you. I will see you in a week. I did my part, now you do yours." And with that, he smiled, waved, turned and left. What a great guy!

"Wow", I thought, "I can go home and to think, no one was sure I would even make it." Remarkable! Later as I went to put on my coat, I gathered my belongings, and thanked all the wonderful people who worked so hard on my behalf. Little did I know, that the hardest part for me was still yet to come.

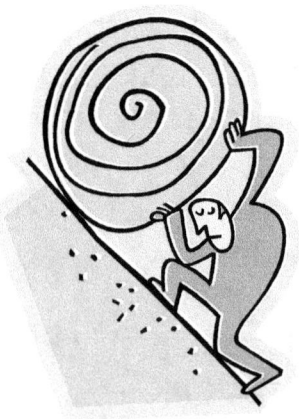

SOME THINGS YOU CAN EXPECT

*Wonderful caring people who are the best at what they do, working very hard to make you better.

* Uncertainness, confusion, some pain, some discomfort, bewilderment. Certainly not feeling well.

* Worry! Grief! Questions that cannot be totally answered yet. (BUT THEY WILL)

* Pills, tubes, and suckie toys.

* Gowns that are open in the back so your butt hangs out!

* Cold floors.

* Lots of people looking all over you.

* Things you want that you cannot have and things you have that you don't want!

* Lots of people asking you lots of questions- sometimes over and over again.

*Food, clothes, and lodging.

*Being waited on hand and foot .

WHAT YOU WILL ACTUALLY GET
*Wonderful caring people who truly care about their patients,

* A dedicated team to monitor your condition, pain, well-being, physical and emotional status.

* HELP AROUND THE CLOCK.

* Gowns that open in the back letting your butt hang out.

* Cold floors, but many warm hearts.

* The comfort that you are on the road to recovery, in the best place that you can be, getting the best of care that is available to you.

* Knowing you will have dedicated long term care when and if you need it.

*Every resource available to make you comfortable on your road to recovery.

WHAT YOU CAN DO TO GET BETTER.
* Listen to what is told to you. If you do not understand, just say so. Have things explained so you <u>do</u> understand.

* Do what is asked of you- even if you don't feel like it. The doctors and nurses only want to help you succeed in getting well.

* Try not to be a grump. It is hard, but your cardiac team will understand up to a point. Everyone has a bad day. Do not be afraid to say you're sorry. That alone will make you feel better.

* Lean on your God, your family and your friends. The ones who love you will support you.

* Give thanks every day for a new beginning.

* When you are troubled, seek and get help. Do not be afraid to ask for help. The resources are there for you.

*And most of all remember... YOU ARE NOT ALONE.   Thousands of people world-wide are going through what you are: young and old, healthy and sickly. You are not the only one. Help others. Let them help you and continue to work hard on getting better. You are the one in control now! It's up to you.

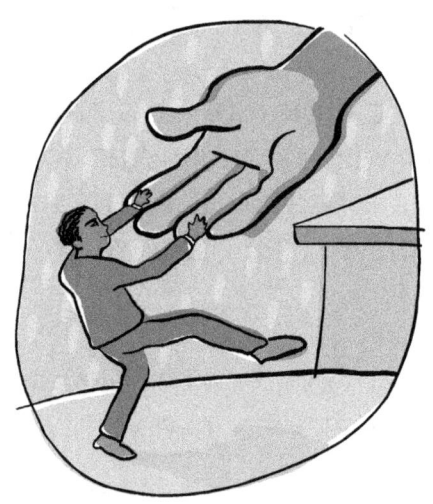

YOUR ATTITUDE

Your attitude will play a major part in your recovery and healing. Whether you have open heart surgery, a heart attack, a valve replacement, a stent, other cardio-vascular issues, a stroke- whatever your problem, we have something in common, we survived. You are now forever changed and all the great doctors in the world and all the best medicines money can buy and all the wonderful people along the way on your road to recovery won't mean a thing if you don't care enough about yourself to get better. So do your part. It is not easy, but it gets easier as you go along. If you want to heal and get better even with a setback now and then, (and they may come along) you and only you can make the decision to get better.

FEELING DISCOURAGED AND BLUE

You may feel sad, lonely, hurt, angry, depressed, anxious, tired, unable to go on, or mad as hell. You may wonder, "Why me?" These feelings are normal. After talking with my fellow patients and looking at my own feelings, I learned that it's okay to feel these emotions. Tell your health care providers and your doctor what you are feeling. They can help you! Remember, you never have to go through these mixed emotions alone. There are many, many people who care. Just speak up. Every day gets a little better. Remember you just had a scary life changing event and a lot of the outcome rests on you.

GET UP & GET MOVING

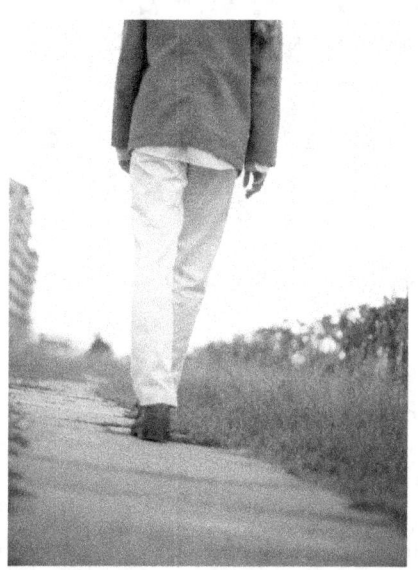

So get up! Get moving! Get help! Welcome to a better tomorrow. You have just been given a second chance at life. Don't waste it. Make the best of it every single day. YOU MY FRIENDS ARE STRONG AND YOU CAN DO THIS! Use every resource available to you and enjoy your new day and the wonderful blessings that are in it.

LITTLE THINGS THAT I LEARNED DURING MY HOSPITAL STAY...

Here are a few things you probably should <u>not</u> take to the hospital should you go:

- Your golf clubs, tennis racket, or YOGA mat
- A six pack of Beer or Soda
- The family Dog
- Twinkies
- Grandma's homemade chili (although it could be comical if you ate some the night before)
- Two or Three Changes of Clothes
- Super Mario Bros
- Drums
- The game OPERATION
- An instructional video on the procedure you are about to have.
- Reference forms for the doctors and nurses to fill out

LEAVE THESE THINGS HOME AS WELL

* Your office Christmas Party

* Hair Dryer

* Cookbook

* Chicken Pot Pies

* Tweetie Bird

* A plunger

* Your own TV

* Ribs, BBQ sauce

and the portable

Grill

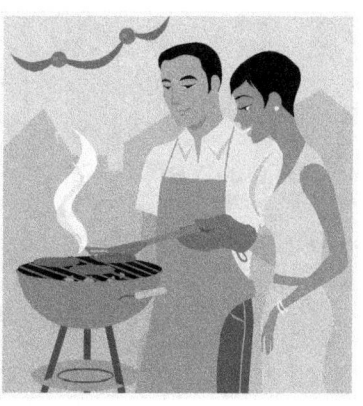

* Your own disinfectant

THINGS YOU SHOULD TAKE SHOULD YOU GO TO THE HOSPITAL

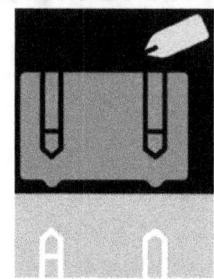

- Yourself
- A complete List of all your 'meds'
- A Driver
- All your medical and insurance (or other) information
- A Positive attitude
- A Smile Helps
- Very few personal products
- A pair of Jammie's and robe with slippers
- A good book

THINGS YOU SHOULD NOT ASK OR SAY DURING AN EXAM OR BEFORE SURGERY

- The instructions are written on my butt.
- Is this your first day?
- I want to see your medical degree along with your grades!
- Is this your second job?
- Do your parents know where you are?
- Aren't you awfully young?
- Are you getting ready to retire?
- Didn't I arrest you for speeding last year?
- Which hallway do we use for the wheelchair races?
- My car is double parked by ER. Can you make sure it doesn't get towed?
- Rest assured, you will get the same top of the line quality care, but you may not make any new friends.

EXPECT THE UNEXPECTED

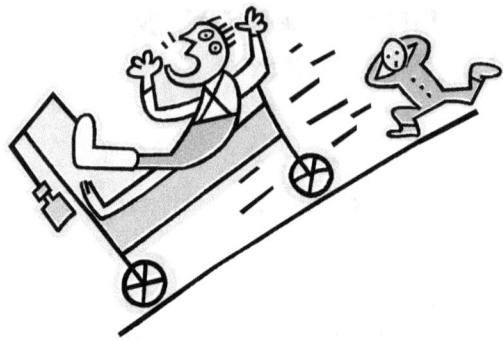

*   Being shaved in places far from the surgical site.

*   Being painted with some kind of antibiotic soap. Mine was blue!

*   Being asked the same questions 187 times within a 20 minute period by four different people.

*   Finding out that the bed pans seem much colder at night.

*   All kinds of people will come running to you should you pull the wrong cord. This is NOT advised.

* Asked who the President of the United States is and "Do you know what day today is?"

* Your fluids going in and coming out being measured.

* Being asked, "How do you feel?" over and over and finding out after thinking about it - not as bad as you first thought.

* Finding out that people really do care about you and how you feel.

* That the food really isn't as bad as its reputation (well maybe once in a while).

* Finding out the bed pans are cold in the day too.

* Your visitors will arrive just as you have fallen asleep.

* Your pills will arrive just as you have fallen asleep.

- You will have to pee just as you are going to sleep or just as you have gotten back in bed.

- The first walk feels a lot longer than it looks.

- Your first REAL bathroom moment (let's leave this one a surprise shall we).

- You will be asked your name and date of birth a LOT!

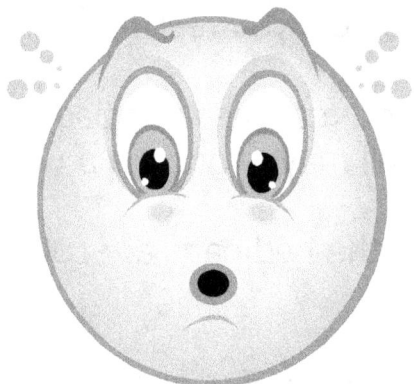

Things You Should expect

A team of dedicated professionals there just for you.

A lot of concern about you, your feelings, and your care.

Information explained to you and should you not understand, explained again in a way you **do** understand.

A commitment to the very best of care possible.

A little work on your part giving all the possible information that you can and doing what is asked of you to help with your recovery

GREAT TV RECEPTION!

People spoiling you a little bit.

Your visitors arriving just as you have fallen asleep.

Cold bed pans (A SORRY FACT, BUT TRUE.)

Clean surroundings with friendly, helpful people.

Your 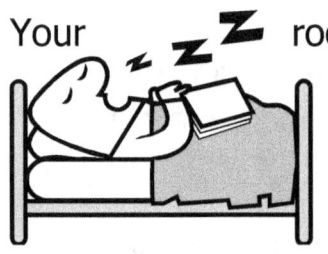 roommate regardless of gender will SNORE like a chainsaw.

Your roommate will say the same about you to his friends. (BET ON THIS ONE)

Quality care with a variety of health care professionals working around the clock for a better tomorrow for ALL THEIR PATIENTS!

Help with forms and payment options Visiting Nursing Service and extended care, if needed, after you go home.

Answers to questions about meds.

People who will listen and address any issues that you may have.

The guidance for your continued well-being.
Follow-up calls to see how you are doing.

Making of new friendships.

And a healthier you!

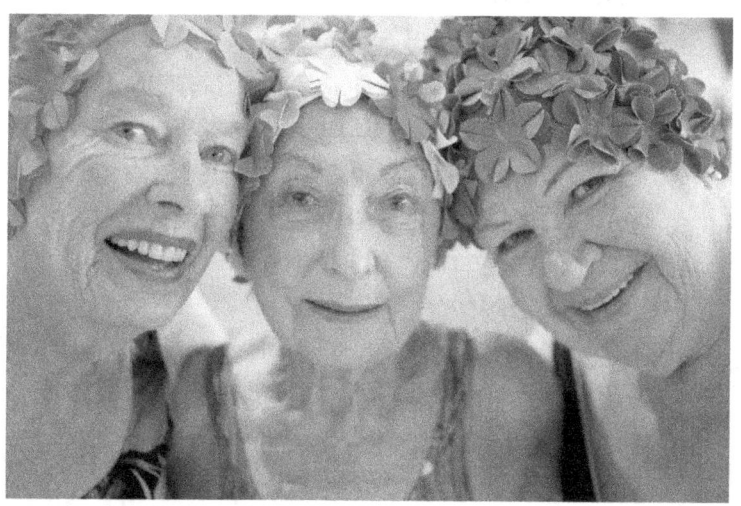

THINGS YOU SHOULD DO UPON LEAVING

- Say Thank You!
- Follow-up with appointments.
- Double check your belongings so you don't forget anything.
- Pass the word about cold bed pans.
- Listen closely to all instructions given and follow them.
- Don't overdo it.
- If you have any questions, now is the time to ask.
- Let your healthcare providers know where you are staying.
- Any concerns? Address them NOW!
- Say Thank You!
- Keep the funny get well cards. Oh what the heck, keep them all.
- Do not ask for a "doggie bag" to take home any removed parts.
- Do something nice for someone else!

GET BETTER...

BE WELL..

HAPPY HEALING!

SAY THANK YOU!

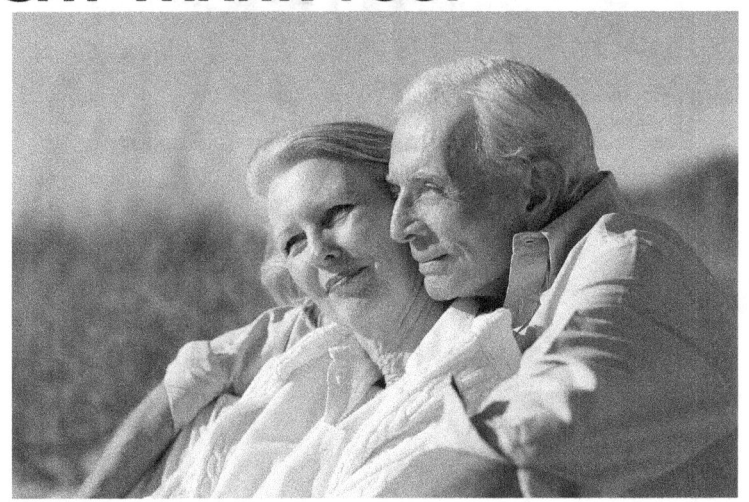

HEADING HOME

Home, Sweet Home

HEADING HOME

Well I'm finally out of the hospital and heading home. It is a cold November evening and I have a 35 minute ride, but it's nice to be out. I arrived home and got settled in. The huggie pillow helps. I am not sure why, but it sure feels good.

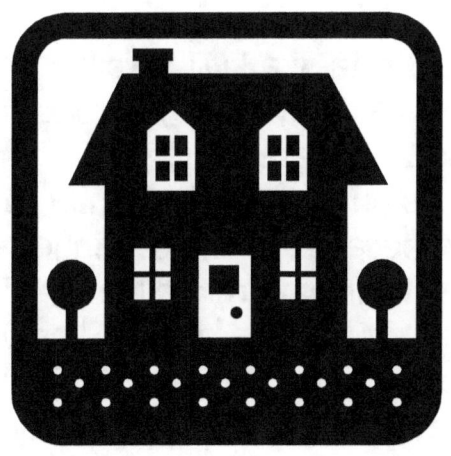

PILLS

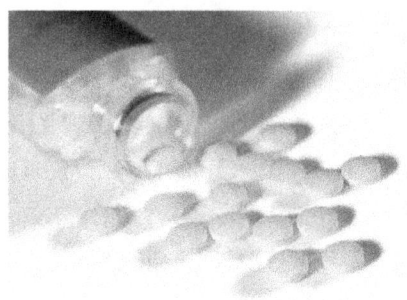

Be prepared to take a LOT of pills. I am not really sure what they all do but back at home I had 27 different pills, all different sizes, shapes and colors that I had to take daily. Now because of my continued improvement through rehabilitation, I only have to take four pills a day.   I know now that they are for a number of GOOD reasons such as preventing clots, keeping you slowed down so you can heal, blood pressure and cholesterol meds just to name a few. The important thing is to take what is prescribed for you. All your prescribed medications play a huge part in your recovery.

THE VISITING NURSE

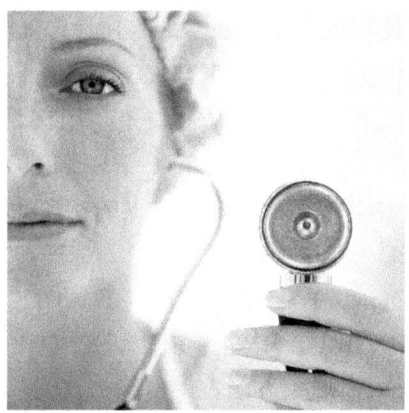

The visiting nurse came before bedtime and checked me over said I looked great. Wow. I think her glasses were dirty, but it was nice to hear. I felt tired and wrung out, but didn't feel a lot of pain, just some discomfort. And it sure felt good to be in my own bed.

AN UNSETTLING SETBACK

Saturday morning I got up and took the mass of pills and decided to walk around as much as I could. Everyone is different and I wanted back to the old me as soon as possible. Funny though, I was told, "You will get tired a lot, your body needs rest to heal and you certainly do not want to overdo it." Wish I had followed this advice! I hope you will learn from my mistakes.

I rested Saturday, but Saturday night it snowed. So Sunday morning, I got up, dressed warm and got on my tractor to plow snow. Well fifteen minutes later, I realized that was a BIG mistake. The cold and the bouncing gave me a reality check in a hurry and as I was slowly heading back in the house the nurse pulled in to my driveway and putting it mildly, gave me a real butt chewing.

 "You are supposed to rest and not exert yourself, lift pull, push, etc., so you don't tear everything apart that they just put back together. That little stunt of yours, Mister, could have caused you a major setback. What were you thinking?"

I meekly answered, "Evidently, I wasn't" Like a scolded dog, I shuffled back into the house with my tail between my legs.

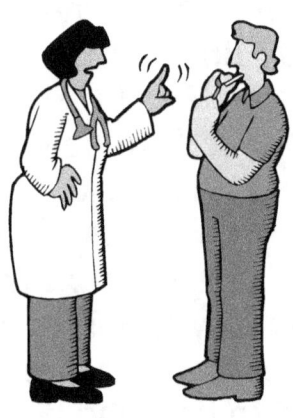

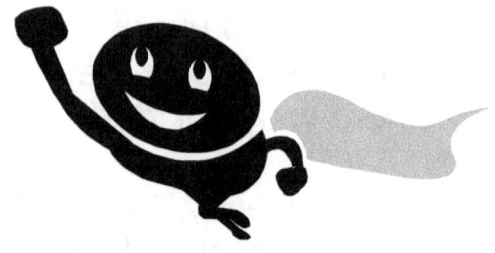

YOU ARE NOT SUPERMAN
....OR WONDER WOMAN

Hey, what she said makes a lot of sense! Hello? Here I was thinking that I was fixed and ready to go. But I pushed myself way too hard. So remember, it takes WEEKS and MONTHS for your body to heal. You have lots of stitches and wire holding your breast bone together. Who knows? Maybe even a little duck tape. Just kidding. I use it for everything. You may feel like you can resume your everyday activities, but hold back! You need to heal and healing takes time. I almost screwed up all that was done because I was not following my doctor's orders. Don't make the same mistake I did.

You may notice that you get cold, and that you bruise easily especially on your arms. Don't worry, it happens from time to time.

94

You are now getting quality blood flow and are probably on a blood thinner, so not to worry. If you have any questions, don't forget to consult you healthcare provider.

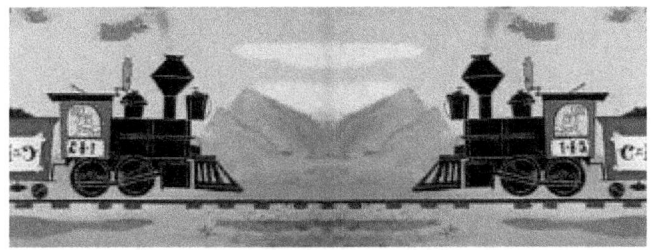

THE TRAIN WRECK
I couldn't wait for band practice! You see I am a singer and a guitar player in a couple of bands. Now twenty sessions into my rehab, I was feeling well enough to start practicing again. I had some speech issues-small ones after my surgery, but overall, I was feeling good and ready to start back up. I was excited. The gang all came over for our first practice. After setting everything up, I was ready to rock and roll. With our guitars on and all tuned up, we started to play and I started to sing some of the songs I have always sung. I was shocked. "What

the heck was that??"   It sounded terrible and everyone was looking at me with a puzzled look on their faces. I stopped the song and then I said, "Okay. Let's start again."

So we started another song and Holy Mackerel, it was awful. Then it hit me. That was **my** voice. It was my singing that sounded so terrible.

Someone said, "Well, it has been awhile. Let's try a slower, softer song."

So "take three." Here I go. It my friends, was a complete train-wreck. I could not sing or control my pitch. My range was gone. I was flat or sharp and sounded terrible on every song I tried. I couldn't sing. I was ***devastated.*** I just couldn't believe it.

The Band was great and everyone told me "Take it easy Steve. We (Cynthia, Erik, and Fred that is,) can take turns singing (THEY ARE ALL GOOD SINGERS) and you can play along for now."

Okay. At the end of the rehearsal, I tried another song. It was the worst yet. I felt defeated, downhearted, and ready to cry.

READY TO QUIT
I said. "I quit. I am tired, sore, angry and just plain devastated. I have been a singer for many years and I really enjoyed and took pride in that and if that is gone, I don't want to continue. I might as well just sell my stuff, pack it in, and stop playing all together." I just was so discouraged and at the end of my rope.

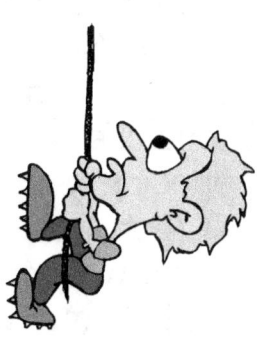

NO QUITTING ALLOWED

"OH NO. YOU'RE NOT GONNA QUIT!" They said it almost at the same moment. Pete, Fred, Cynthia, Erik, and Jay all said, "We will work with you and stand by you till you figure out what is going on. You may need extra help so go and see a throat doctor and find out what's up with you. We will support and help you." What a great bunch of folks!

AFTER THE TRAIN WRECK

Well I couldn't' sing anymore but my band friends told me to get help. So I thought, "Okay, let's give it a shot." I made a doctor's appointment with an ENT (Ear, Nose and Throat) specialist to see what was going on and what could be done to help me with this issue. After examining me, he suggested a complete throat and esophageal exam. This involved a tiny camera on a small flexible kind of wire (tube). I'm not sure what to call it. It was inserted down my throat. It didn't really hurt, but it was a bit uncomfortable.

WHAT WAS HAPPENING IN MY THROAT

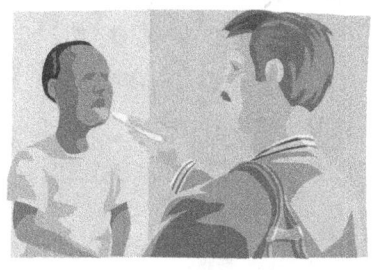 The doc took photos and didn't see any obvious signs of disease. He suggested that I try Speech Therapy. He explained what was going on with my throat in layman's terms. He said that I had irritation and swelling in and around my voice box and some stress and strains involving the control of the diaphragm and vocal chords. Apparently some of the tubes that helped saved my life, along with the trauma of being paddled (shocked) a couple times, played a part in the problems that I was experiencing right then.

MOVING FORWARD

I was given some tips on how important is to drink LOTS OF WATER to keep my throat and voice box hydrated. The doctor also gave me a prescription for some nasal spray to help with allergies that I was experiencing and scheduled a follow- up exam two weeks later. I promised him that I would call Speech Therapy and make an appointment to see the speech therapist ASAP, which I did.

MY APPOINTMENT WITH THE SPEECH THERAPISTS

The day of my appointment, I had no clue as what to expect. I met with two ladies who did the examination and scoped my throat again. They involved the doctor whom I had just seen days earlier and together planned what to do to help me. They also gave me a microphone and had me talk and sing. They had me go from the lowest note in my register to the highest note that I was able to make. It was pretty cool. A computer recorded and actually charted out what I did. I guessed that the data could be analyzed and retained for comparison purposes later. Anyway, it was neat. They were really nice and very understanding, extremely knowledgeable and charted the course for my treatments.

MY SESSIONS
I scheduled my sessions somewhat apprehensively and wondered what would happen over the next few weeks. I was recorded. I was given voice exercises to do. I learned a lot about my voice, about speech, about how sounds are made and formed, and about the role of the vocal chords.

ON A SIDE NOTE
On a side note, my vocal chords looked neat when they were forming a sound. It was definitely pretty cool to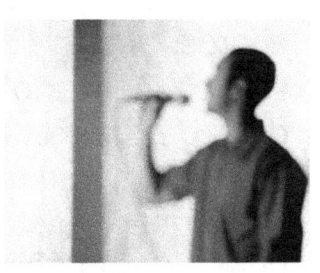
see. Sometimes, I laid on the floor while doing vocal exercises. Sometimes, they had

me doing exercises while standing or sitting. All the time, I was being monitored and encouraged. I learned about breathing, about foods, and how hot and cold drinks have an affect on the vocal chords and throat. I also learned about the effects of a cold, sinus and ear infections, allergies and never really realized how all these things could affect your voice.

I was tested and my progress was charted and analyzed each visit, I also had regular visits with the ENT doctor to follow my progress.

LESSONS LEARNED

I learned a lot about the importance of water and hydration of the throat, the vocal chords, and the body. I learned how to reduce the risk of straining, and the damage that could occur from yelling, screaming, and, smoking. I also was taught the proper way to form and phrase words, notes, sounds, pronunciation and proper breathing. You never really think about all that is involved in being able to speak a single word or sing one note. It is amazing what transpires when you speak or sing. There are a lot of things all going on inside you just to make a simple sound. Wow.

THE GIFT OF SINGING AGAIN
The specialists who treated me and continued to encourage me all through my sessions were the best. I mean this.   What a gift they gave to me.   They made it possible for me to go back to singing again. That along with the support of my fellow musicians, was to say the very least, overwhelming at times and very humbling. I continued treatments for weeks and still have checkups and follow-ups on a regular basis with my ENT doctor and the speech pathologist.

GRATITUDE

I also am so grateful for the time and extra patience that they showered me with. I was very discouraged when I started and for a few weeks, I was not very optimistic. But as things started to improve, so did my spirits. And all I can say is to them is "Thank you so much!"

SPEECH ISSUES: NO BOUNDARIES

I also found that speech and throat issues know no boundaries. Although the sessions that I attended were one on one, I also witnessed and met other patients from toddlers and little children to young adults and older seasoned people like myself. All were experiencing some kind of issue and the care that we all received was outstanding in every sense of the word.

WHO WOULD HAVE KNOWN?

I never realized the complex and many different throat, ear, nose, and speech issues that there are, not to mention, the complications of disease, strokes, injury, birth defects. Wow. There are so many different and complex issues that can arise and most of us never give a second thought to them. Until I met others with speech issues, and their caregivers, I simply had no idea what folks deal with on a daily basis. My hat is off to you, folks.

SINGING AGAIN

So I am singing again and am raising funds for my favorite charities. I am also speaking better. I am very thankful for the wonderful people who pushed me to do better and encouraged me every step of the way. Sharing their expert advice, while working hard have helped me and others like me to get better and lead a higher quality of life every day. Not only are they great at what they do, they are the best in their given professions and I am so humbled and proud to say that they now are also my friends, whom I cherish, respect and value each and every day.

SEEK ADVICE!

As with any problem. if you have any throat, ear, nose, sinus, or speech issues, please seek medical help and advice NOW!!! Yes, seek and get help right away. Do not wait. In a medical emergency, call 911 immediately. Do not hesitate, you have a voice! Be heard and do not take it for granted. Take care of yourself, please.

SETBACKS

Also remember that a setback can happen to any of us at any time, but if you approach it as a challenge and seek out help, if you work hard and listen to the advice given you, the better your chances are for a good outcome. So at times during my journey to wellness, I attended two different rehabilitation programs: Cardio Rehab and Speech Rehab. I also had numerous doctor visits with my primary doctor, my cardiologist and my new ENT doctor. Looking back, it's no wonder I needed a nap!

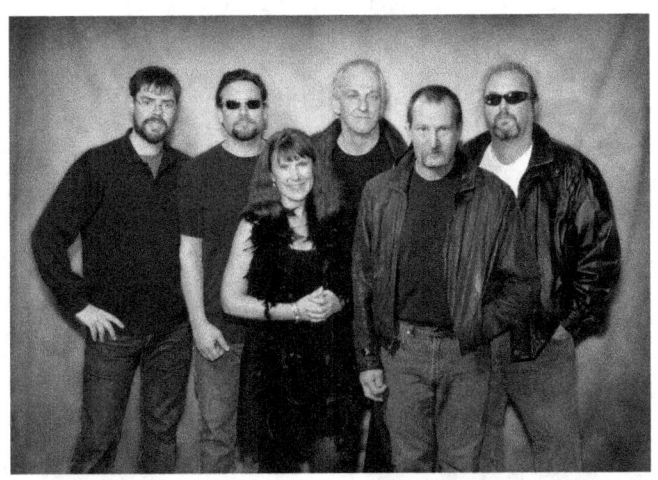

Here's a photo of the band (at the time). What a great group of friends. Left to right: Jay Palmer, Fred DeBuck, Cynthia Huling Hummel, me, Erik Will and Pete Kitchen. (photo courtesy of Jay Palmer Photography)

A GOOD DECISION

I'm so glad that I made the decision to go to a throat doctor who not only diagnosed my problem but also referred me to speech therapy, which ultimately made it possible for me to sing again. But at that time, I was not happy nor was I confident that it would make a difference. I was not only discouraged, I was ashamed to tell anyone I was having trouble with my voice. But I decided to give speech therapy a go. Wow, was I glad that I did. After weeks of working on speaking and voice exercises, my voice started to come back. Yep, with a little hard work and a lot of patient, caring people who worked hard to help me overcome this little setback, I was getting better.

A SIDE NOTE

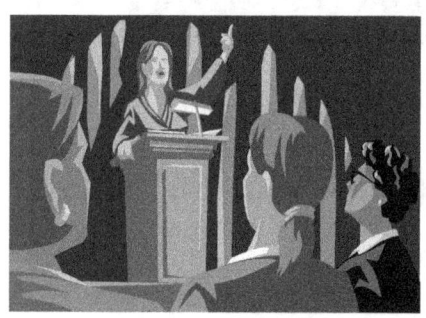 As a side note, I also joined Toastmasters International, which is an organization with clubs worldwide, that help you become the speaker that you always wanted to be.   The club that I belong to is a GREAT club with wonderful people who guide each other to become better public speakers while building confidence and offering constructive guidance.   I strongly recommend Toastmasters to anyone and everyone.

DON'T GIVE UP

By the grace of God and with the help of a great band, I slowly started to get my voice back. I started singing easy mellow songs and after a couple months, I was back to belting out songs with the best of them. My band buddies said that I sounded better and stronger than ever. The point I am trying to make is that you may experience a setback from time to time and if you do, *DON'T GIVE UP.*

As tough as it can be at times, seek the help that you need to get through it, and to continue to get better. It sometimes seems easier to quit and you may have already been through a lot but in all honesty, you can do it. The effort is well worth the reward. Just like Cardio Rehab and life, until you try, you never know how far you can go. And should you stumble, learn from it and keep going! A little setback is just what it says it is a LITTLE setback, that's all. Your road to recovery depends mostly on how you drive it. You are in control. Take the wheel.

FINDING COMFORT

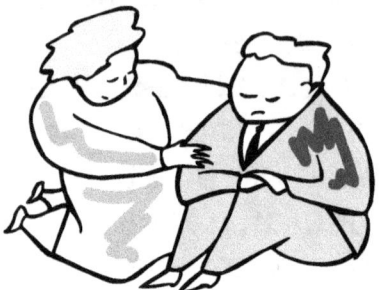

How do you find comfort?   For me, it included talking about how I felt. It also helped to have a Prayer Shawl, given to me by some folks at a church. I wrapped myself up and found great comfort knowing so many people cared and were praying for me. Some I did not even know. Remember, many people care about you. Take the time to notice them.

Take some downtime and read up on what exactly was done. Educate yourself about your procedure. This will help you understand what you went through, what to expect and how to cope and continue to get yourself better.

FOLLOW-UP!

Go to your follow-up appointments. Tell your visiting nurse of any problems and as the pills slowly get backed off, you may start feeling better. It's time to start looking ahead to cardio rehabilitation. More likely than not, your team of doctors will want you to attend cardio rehab and that is something YOU SHOULD DO!!!!! I repeat YOU NEED IT. YOU WILL BENEFIT FROM IT <u>and</u> you will be glad that you did.

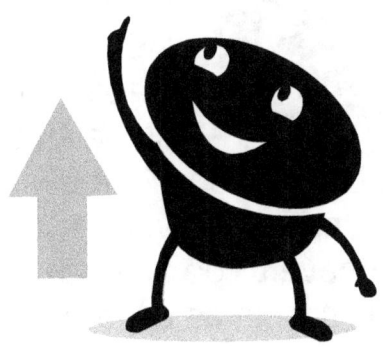

FAITH, FRIENDS , FAMILY AND YOU

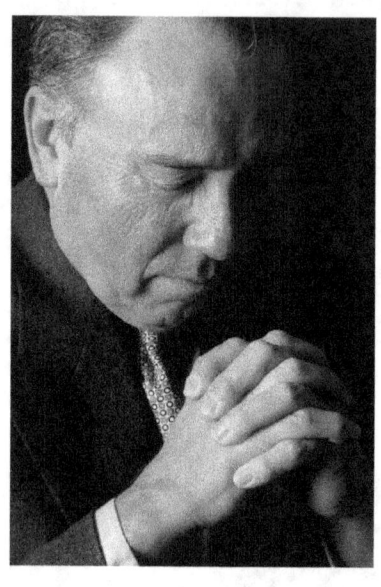

No matter what your faith is or feelings are, we all carry hidden strengths that help us in troubled times. And we often pray for help. I call on God to give me the strength and guidance to carry on when I am troubled. Whatever it is that you believe in, make that spiritual connection. Your own personal faith will do a lot to help you in your time of need. All you have to do is reach out. If your condition is as simple as controlling high blood pressure or as serious as a heart transplant, you have your inner strength to draw on. Use it. Your own faith, determination, will, and positive mindset can be great assets to you in the days to come.

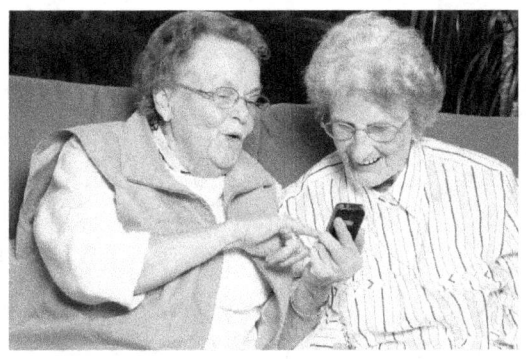

LEAN ON YOUR FRIENDS.

We all have friends. Some are close and others are distant. Some are just "fair-weather" friends. Some we just love and some we tolerate. Your friends can be a great help to you in your recovery and journey to wellness. If you cannot drive yet, perhaps a friend could drive you to an appointment. Should you find that it is harder for you to do certain things that you used to do, call on a friend for a hand. Your friends can help boost your spirits, bring a smile, and give a listening ear when you feel the need to just talk.

PICK UP THE PHONE AND CALL A FRIEND

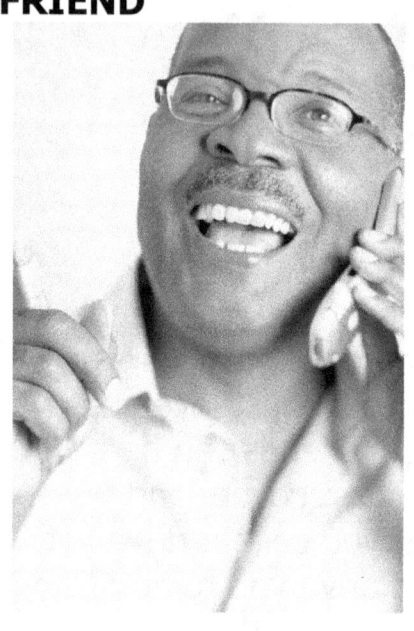

You know who you can call on in times of need and who will be there in a heartbeat should you need help!   So if people want and offer to help you, by all means, take them up on it. Just as you would go and help a friend with no hesitation, call them. Often times when we need a hand, we don't want to bother anyone and we try to go it alone when people are waiting and wanting to help us. So just ask. Your friends will be there for you. Let them help if they can.

KEEP YOUR FAMILY IN THE LOOP

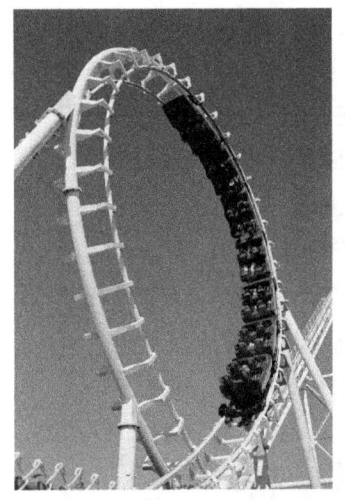 As with all families, some are very close and some may be scattered about. Explain what is happening and how you feel to your family. Remember they are concerned about you and want to help and they also may not realize or understand exactly what your condition is, what may be involved, how you feel physically, and what is on your mind. They may not understand that it is harder for you now to do certain things that you used to do and that you don't feel up to doing some things. Speak up. Keep them in the loop.

CONFIDENCE

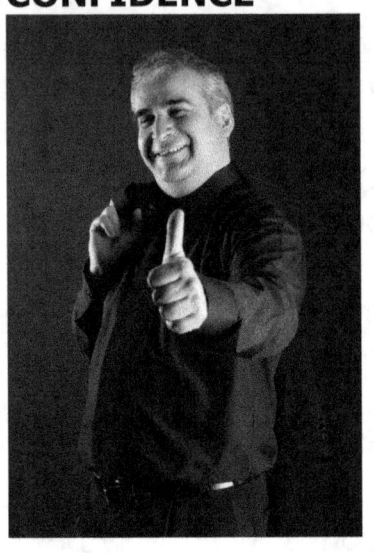

Some say that confidence is having a trust or faith in a person or thing. Others say it is the reliability of a person or a thing. What is it that builds confidence? Is it doing something over and over? Is it something you are born with? Is it a feeling of self-worth? Or might it be more about self-image, success, or how others perceive you?

To me, confidence and self-confidence are like a baby taking its first steps. They are small steps, while holding on to a finger. At some point, the baby realizes that the finger isn't there any more and that he did it: he walked by himself. With that comes the look: happy, laughing, scared, and sometimes the baby falls flat in his butt. It is the small steps that build confidence.

Confidence is something that some have too little of and others seem to have too much of. One thing that we all have in common, is that we need confidence in life. It is like the air we breathe. We need it to survive. We need to achieve and to grow as individuals. Without confidence, we cannot continue on our journey to wellness.

JUST BE YOURSELF

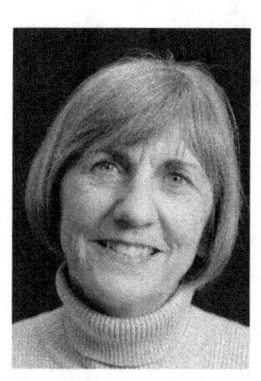 As individuals, we are often trying to live up to other people's expectations of us and at the same time, trying to live up to our own expectations of ourselves. Sometimes we succeed and sometimes, we do not. The one thing that we sometimes forget is to be ourselves and just to improve who and what we are- not for anyone else- but for ourselves.

Confidence sometimes get confused with conceit, arrogance, cockiness, self-centeredness and I suppose that at times, they do spill over into one another.

A CONFIDENT PERSON STANDS OUT

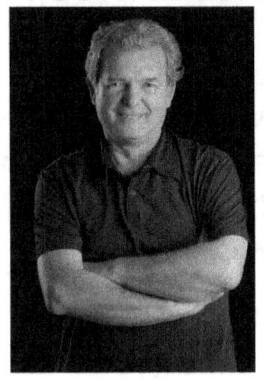

Yes, a truly confident person stands out, not as conceited or arrogant, but as a leader who builds confidence within others and directs their energy to the potential not the limitations- to the possibilities, not the difficulties- and to the fact that they themselves know their limitations, but are not afraid to reach a little higher.

Learning, sharing, practice, participation, the ability to laugh at yourself and understanding that you do have flaws, that you can handle rejection, and that you will not always be perfect, are small baby steps in building confidence.

In letting go of the fingers that hold us all back as we take our baby steps will enable each of us to gain self-worth, self-esteem, and help us grow our self-confidence as we continue to invest and reinvest in ourselves, learning from our stumbles and falls and facing the challenges ahead from the confidence that continues to grow with us every day.

GROWING IN CONFIDENCE

Think of confidence as a baby learning to walk and taking those first few steps as time goes on. With practice, patience and the inner strength that we all possess, and by building on our own individual strengths while recognizing our weaknesses, with each step that we take, our confidence will grow also. Confidence knows no age or barrier. But it does need nurturing, guidance, and thrives for new learning experiences to grow and mature just like you and I.

CONFIDENCE: THE FUEL IN YOUR TANK

Your wanting to grow, excel, learn, succeed, and prosper are all signs of your confidence driving you to be the best that you can be. Confidence is like fuel in your tank. Your ability to drive yourself to be the leader that you want to be or have the confidence in others, that make a difference in people's lives every day, while they share and instill confidence in you. No box to think out of here. Dare to be different. A box only holds so much and can be a cage. Walk your own mile. Follow your own dreams and let confidence take you to your goal of wellness.
YOU CAN DO IT.

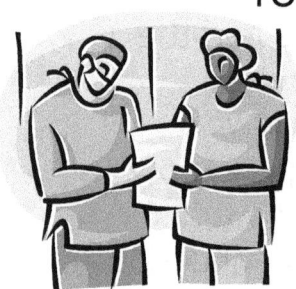

HAVE CONFIDENCE IN YOUR TEAM

Have confidence in your journey to wellness and in all the people who are helping along the way: your doctors, nurses, therapists, technicians, dieticians, etc. These folks are your wellness team. Have confidence in them and in yourself. You can do this and you are not alone.

COMMUNICATION IS THE KEY

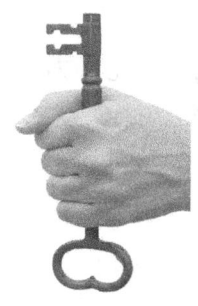

Communication is the key to everyone understanding why you are making the decisions that you are and why some days you just do not feel like doing something that others may want to do. They need to know your concerns and they also need to know what your condition is, the treatments involved and that you may need moral and physical support. The better you communicate your concerns and the better they communicate their concerns or questions, the better it will be for all parties involved. Brainstorm with each other on what is best for you and them.

DO A BETTER JOB: COMMUNICATE!

Although I certainly could have done a better job of communicating with my own family and others, I see now that by trying to do everything myself and by holding everything inside, I did them and myself a disservice and better communication would have benefited all involved. Total communication between you, your doctors, nurses, and family will help everyone better understand what is needed for your well-being.

UNCERTANTIES

You may be worried, unsure and have a lot of questions. You may also be wondering what awaits you in the days to come. We all face uncertainties. We may have lots of questions. Don't worry. It's part of life. We make decisions everyday on what to wear what to have for lunch, which movie to see, but this is different. This affects your health and overall well-being.

If you are uncertain about which road to take in your journey to wellness, ask for directions and guidance to help ease your uncertainties from one or more of the many resources that are available to you.

122

PAY ATTENTION TO YOUR BODY AND ASK QUESTIONS

Pay attention to your body and what it is telling you. Listen to your doctors and healthcare providers. Research your condition and the treatments involved. KNOW AS MUCH ABOUT YOUR CONDITION AND WHAT IS INVOLVED AS YOU POSSIBILY CAN. ASK QUESTIONS AND HAVE THINGS EXPLAINED TO YOU IN TERMS THAT YOU CAN UNDERSTAND. Your will and the ability to deal with your condition depend greatly on your understanding. It is the key.

IT DEPENDS ON YOU

How you feel, questions you may have, treatments available, alternatives, etc., are all things you need to chart your course to a better you. You are in the driver's seat and you hold a lot of the decisions and the expected results in YOUR hands. Many things will come into play here, and much of it, depends on YOU!

So reach out to your faith, your friends, and your family. Always seek medical help and guidance. Take charge of today and move forward to a better tomorrow.

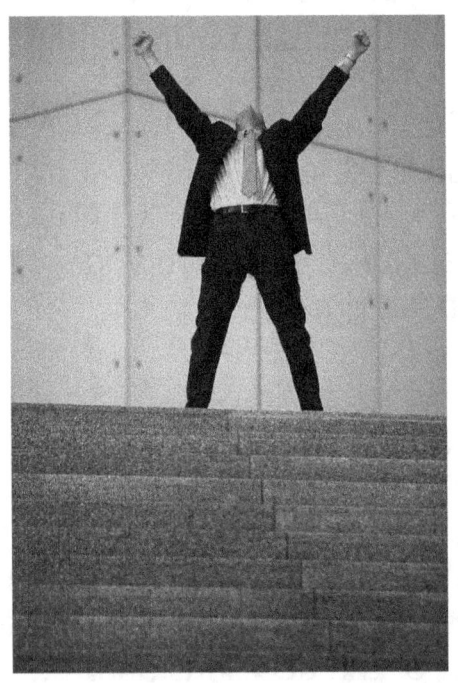

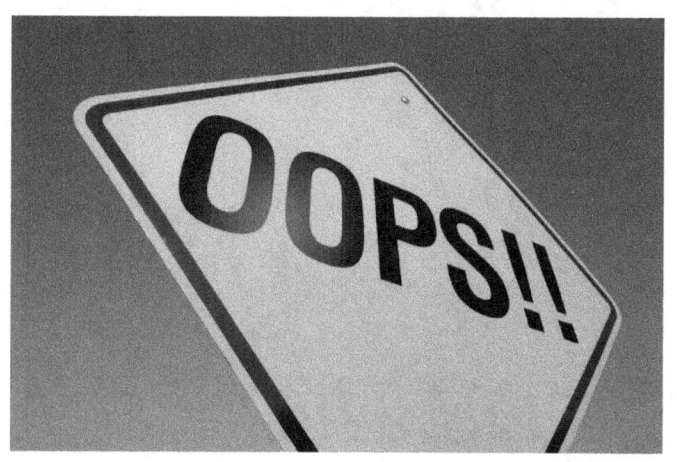

LEARN FROM MY MISTAKES

Don't make some of the same mistakes that I made by trying to go it alone; by not wanting to bother anyone, and by not following the advice that I was given (well, I did a little) Looking back, I should have followed my own advice and the advice offered on a lot of what I have just listed. Now I know better! And every day I am still learning and still healing and still working hard towards a better tomorrow. THIS TIME, IT IS ABOUT YOU!!! Draw on all your resources: THIS TIME IT IS ABOUT YOU!!!

THE THREE PHASES OF CARDIO CARE

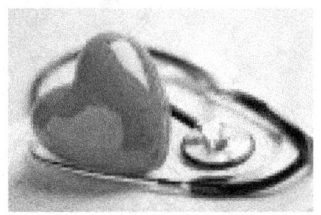

* **Phase One** is the event and correction (such as the surgery or procedures performed.)

* **Phase Two** is being monitored and much needed rehabilitation.

* **Phase Three** is continuing on-going rehabilitation, more or less at your own pace.

You will have many mixed emotions as the time progresses. Some days will feel better than others. This is all normal. You have had a life changing event.

REST EASY

If you are going for treatment or are scheduled for surgery, you can rest easy knowing there is nothing that you cannot handle. The outcome can be far better than the way things are for you now. Given a little time, you will feel better and have a better quality of life for it. So do not hesitate. Consult with your healthcare providers and make the choices that are best for you, based on your current condition.

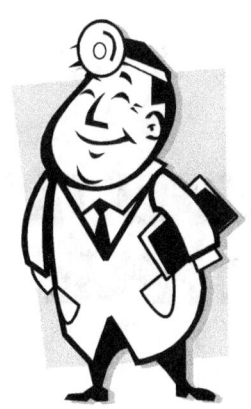

GETTING STRONGER AND FEELING BETTER

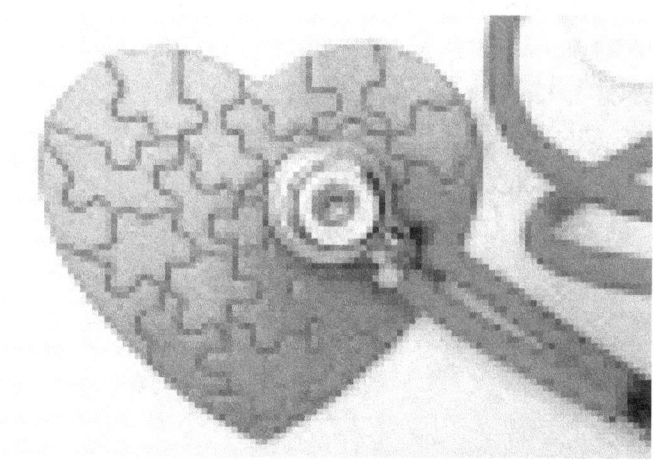

CARDIO- REHABILTATION: THE SECOND PHASE

PHASE 2 CARDIO REHAB

Well by now you are probably leaving Phase One which involved your diagnosis, hospital visit and corrective measures taken by you and your team of health care professionals. Many health care providers will recommend Phase 2 cardio rehab. The program in which I enrolled was for 36 visits. I went three days a week. Your schedule and program will be tailored to your doctor's recommendations. You may be a little apprehensive. Well don't be shy or scared! This will be one of the best things you have ever done for yourself.

NO SECRETS OR SHORTCUTS

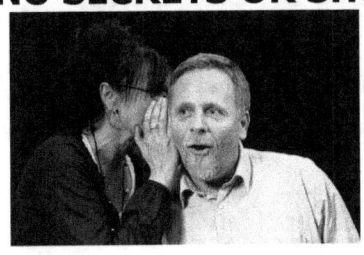 There are no secrets or shortcuts to cardio rehab. You will get out exactly what you put into it and you will benefit greatly from this program. It will be one of the best gifts you have ever given yourself. What a joy to feel better, stronger, more sure and knowledgeable about yourself and your

health. Plus, you will meet new friends, some older, some younger, but all working like you to get healthier. So let's get started.

GETTING STARTED

After you sign up for the Phase 2 Cardio Rehab program, you will be introduced to your nurses who are the best of the best at what they do! They will explain what you will do and the level you will work on. We are all different and some people will workout harder than you and some less. Your doctor and cardiologists will determine what is best for you. You will be weighed and a list of all your medications will be documented. You will have an EKG done which will also be done on a routine basis. You will be shown how to wear "the Box."

THE BOX

The box will monitor your heart rate while you are at cardio-rehab. Your vital signs will be monitored including your pulse and blood pressure. Your heart function, your breathing and your overall performance will be watched closely while you are exercising.

This is to ensure you do not overdo things and that all goes well.

Okay, now we are here, so let's look around the room at what you will see and do. You may notice a chart on the wall that gives guidance on the cardio rehab program.

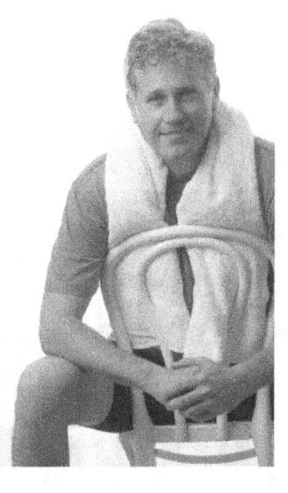

Every session will begin with a warm up and end with cool downs, after which you relax for 5-10 minutes

You will do warm-ups and stretch your arms, legs, neck, etc. You get the picture. (NOTE: after warming up and doing this countless times I still refer to the chart everyday like I am seeing it for the first time.) It's funny! You would think I would know it by now! Hey, I never said I was smart!

HOW DO YOU FEEL WHILE EXERCISING?

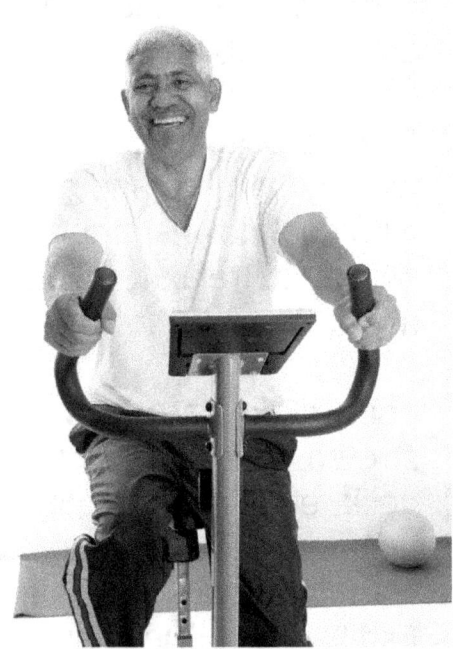

In the cardio rehab program I attended, we refer to a chart that hangs on the wall to describe how we feel when we are exercising. I guess you could say it describes the intensity. I have included my own description in the column to follow.

(These are only my own descriptions and not intended as a guide) The cardio rehab nurses will let you know what you can and CAN'T do based on your doctor's instructions, your progress and your medical statistics.

As you get stronger, you may be allowed to do a bit more. And always, after your workout, you will do cool downs and rest for 5-10 minutes. Your vital signs will be taken again before you leave. If you have any discomfort, during rehab, stop and let the nurses know immediately.

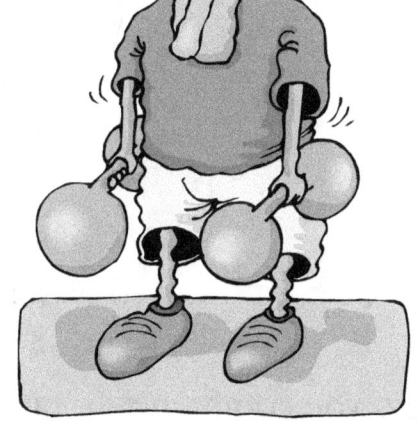

The BORG RPE Chart

Their Chart Definitions	Mine
6 No exercise at all (resting)	Nice! This is easy
7 Extremely light	I can do this sleeping
8	OK. No big deal!
9 Very light	It must be working
10	This is ok, but I can do more
11 Light	Look at me!
	No sweat I'm Golden!
12	whew!
13 Somewhat Hard	Sweating!!
14	a little sweat is OK
15 Hard (heavy)	I can feel this one
16	How much longer?
17 Very hard	Are you kidding me?
18	What are you nuts?
	No way!
19 Extremely hard	Holy Crap! Is this legal?
20 Maximal exertion	Peaked out! I'm done!
	I need a nap!

This chart lets you communicate on how hard or easy it is for you at the time of exercising and also helps your team of nurses track your progress so that you don't overexert yourself. There is more information on the BORG chart at the end of this book. You will use a host of equipment on your road to a better you. I've noted some of the equipment at the Cardio Rehab Center where I go, in the chart that follows.

Equipment Name/ My notes
Arm Exercise machine
    (The Tormentor)
Treadmill
    (Torture Rack)
Rowing machine
    (A Boat trip without water)
Stepping machine
    (No Comment %^$#$)
Stationary bike
    (The Butt Pincher)
Leg and Arm machine
    (Skiing without snow)
Recumbent Bike
    (Bark-o-lounger)
Two step stairs
    (Up & down going nowhere
    while you feel you're going somewhere)
Hand Weights
    (The arm ache-ers)

GETTING STRONGER

All of these machines can help build strength and endurance. The exercises you do will help you build strength and endurance while conditioning your heart, according to the guidelines set by your doctor. As you get stronger, your rate of resistance may increase. Keep at it. You will feel better and have fun doing it. IT ALL TAKES TIME. Don't rush things. Follow instructions. Visit and enjoy as you go. It is all good.

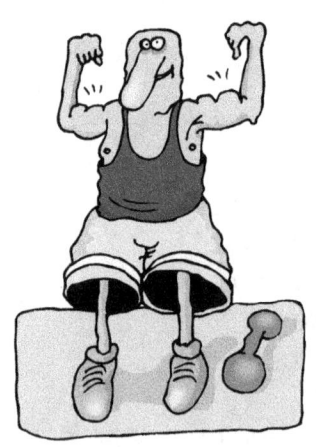

MORE INFORMATION ON GETTING WELL ..... AND STAYING WELL

Your cardio rehab program may be more than an exercise program. Mine was. We also saw instructional videos on nutrition, exercise, cholesterol and heart related information, etc. We got flyers and handouts to read. You see, another goal of the program is to teach cardio patients more about making healthy choices. For example, we learned about good and bad cholesterol, how to make better choices in the foods we eat, how stress affects us, heart health, etc.

DON'T BE AFRAID TO ASK

Take advantage of these information sessions. Ask questions. The more you learn, the better decisions you can make about your heart health. You are on a great journey to a new and improved you, with many people to help you along the way.

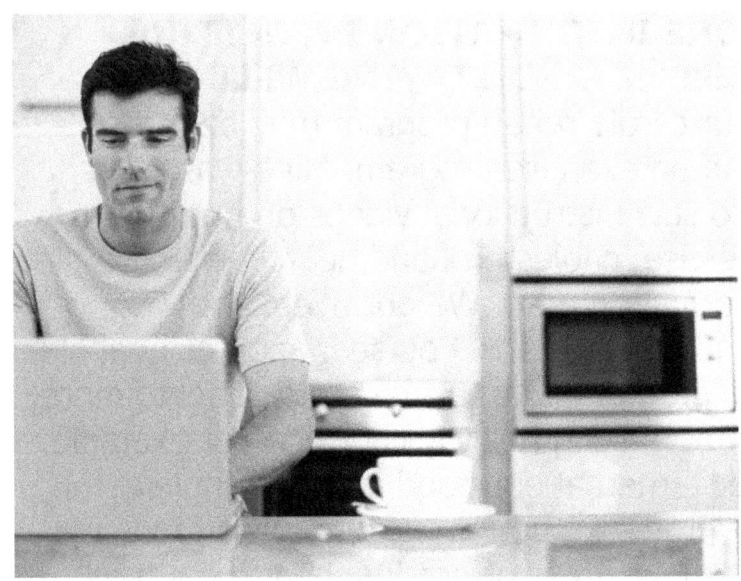

TRANSITIONING BACK TO WORK.
Well by now you and your doctor have
discussed the possibility of your returning to
work, school, or retirement. You feel better
and if you are like me, you are ready to get
back to doing all the things that have been
put on hold. You are changed now. You
have had an event that has forever made an
in impact on your life: big or small, it's still
something to keep an eye on and certainly
follow-up. I was happy to get back to work.
I was out of work from November through
April perhaps even the first week of May.
Some of you may be out only a couple days

or a week, while others like myself, may be out for months or more, depending on your procedure.

When it's time to start resuming normal activities, you may feel better than ever with more energy and much less discomfort or you still may feel weak and tire easily. Whatever the case, I would urge you to NOT OVERDO THINGS!

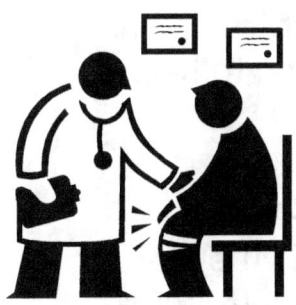 **HAVE A HEART-TO -HEART CHAT WITH YOUR DOCTOR**
Have a heart-to-heart talk with your doctor about what you can and what you should not do. If your job involves heavy lifting or long strenuous hours, high stress, etc., please discuss those concerns with your health care providers. Perhaps you can be temporally transferred to a lighter duty job or you may still need a little more time. Either way, communication is the key.

HEALING TAKES TIME

Your body needs time to heal and you need time to regain your strength and stamina. We are all different. Some heal faster than others, but we all need to pay close attention to what we do and the advice we are given. Many people played a huge role in our treatment and the advice given is only given to help us make a complete recovery.

GETTING WELL TAKES WORK

I urge you to seriously consider on-going exercise and continue rehabilitation: Cardio Phase Three, which we will talk about in a little bit- or consider a doctor guided exercise program. Getting well will take a little work on your part. It's sometimes hard, but it really is for your own good and well-being. Watch your diet, eat healthy, exercise, stop smoking, and please listen to the advice your health care providers offer you. I am not a doctor. I am only a patient like yourself- just sharing my journey with you.

SEEK AND FOLLOW

Always seek and follow medical advice from the professionals who are treating you. And as with anything else, should you have a concern that you feel is not being addressed, seek a second opinion. I resumed work and continued my rehabilitation, not pushing myself as hard as I did before, and with each passing week, I continued to feel better, and get stronger. I realized that I had been given a second chance at life and I was going to try and do better this time around in taking care of myself.

BACK IN THE SADDLE?

A few things you may notice
when you return to work:

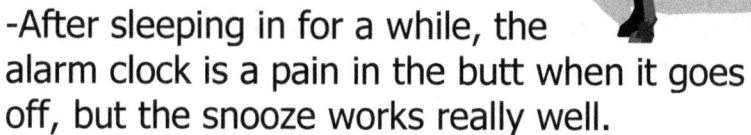

-After sleeping in for a while, the
alarm clock is a pain in the butt when it goes
off, but the snooze works really well.

-An eight hour day feels like a ten hour day
for a while.

-When you get home, you may nap through
the 6 o'clock news.

-You actually feel so much better and it is
sure nice not to have the nagging tightness
in your chest whenever you do something.

-The sky looks a little more blue.

-You will love the comments: "You look
great!"

- It's great to hear that you were missed!

-It feels great to be out of the house and back in the groove!

- If you are retired, you may feel better doing the things that you love to do.

-You are really going to miss the afternoon shows you got used to watching on TV. And after a week back, you may wonder, "Why the heck did I watch that stuff????" (Confession time: I did kind of get hooked on Rachel Ray.)

- Hopefully, you have learned a lot about you and your condition. Use that knowledge every day.

-If you have any problems, issues, questions, etc., talk to your doctor asap!

-Anytime you have any concerns, get help immediately.

-Your body will let you know when something is not right. Listen to it and seek help!

So get up! Get moving, and get started on moving forward with the new you.

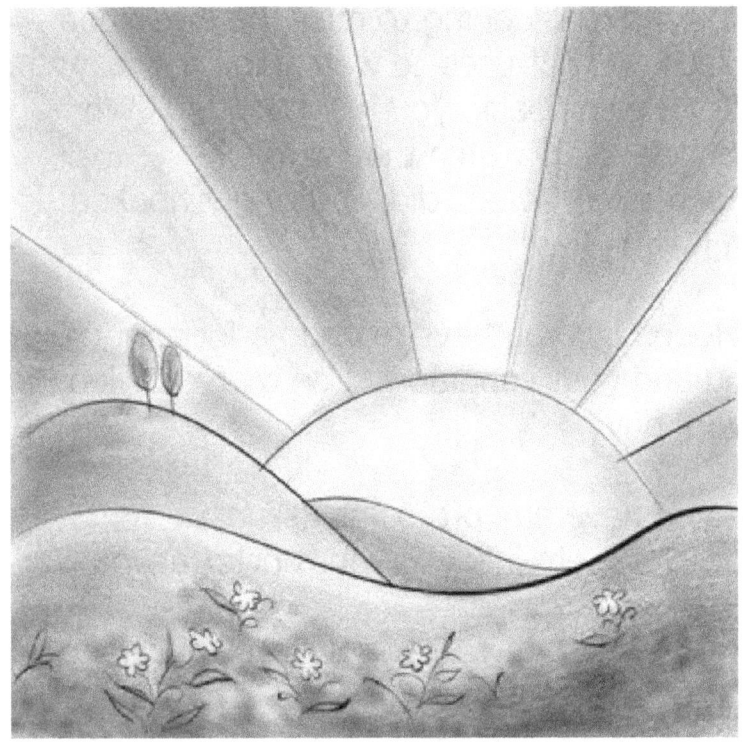

GRADUATION DAY: THE COMPLETION OF CARDIO REHAB PHASE TWO

Well you did it. You have 36 sessions under your belt. Look how far you have come. Good for you. Take a moment and remember how you felt when you started and how you feel now. Be honest. What a nice change. Depending on the facility you may get a certificate, t-shirt or perhaps even a little cake. This is one time you can have your cake and eat it too.

YOU CAN (and should) BE PROUD OF YOURSELF!!

CONGRATULATIONS! YOU DID IT!

Well done. Now you must make a very important decision: to take what you have learned and continue on, or go back to everyday life as it was? Give this some serious thought!! We will talk in a bit about Phase 3.

TAKING THE NEXT STEP:

Okay. Here we are. You have completed Phase Two rehabilitation. Congratulations to you! What a milestone. And now you are more than likely back to a somewhat normal routine, back doing a lot of the things that you enjoy doing (and some you do not.) My question to you is this: What will you do now to continue on your road to recovery?

Some of you will exercise on your own. Some of you will jump back into work full steam ahead, and sadly some of you will do nothing. I STRONGLY recommend that you sign up for ongoing continued cardiac rehabilitation! This folks will be one of the very best gifts that you can give to yourself and those you love.

You already know your caregivers from Phase Two Rehabilitation and some of the people you have attended sessions with. Some may have already moved on to Phase Three Rehab and others are still signing up, but all are working hard to be on the road to a healthier life and you should too!

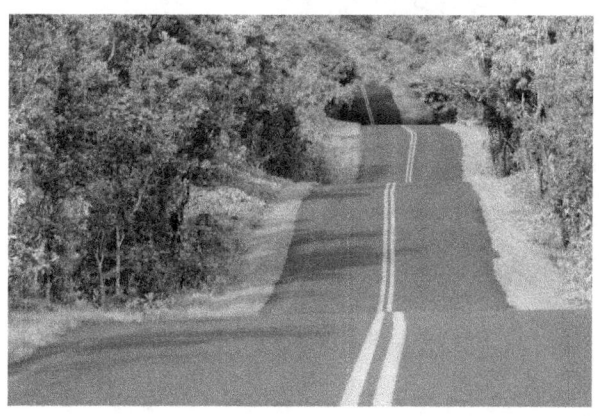

TAKE THE ROAD TO A HEALTHIER YOU!

TAKING THE NEXT STEP ON THE ROAD TO RECOVERY...

CARDIO PHASE THREE

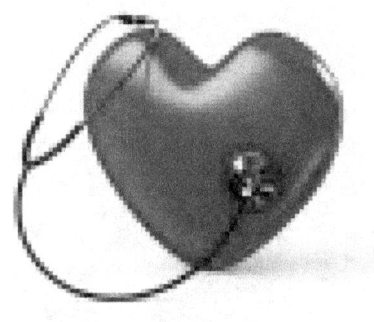

PHASE THREE CARDIO REHAB OR PERSONALIZED ONGOING REHABILITATION

Let me explain a little bit about what is called Phase Three Rehabilitation. In Phase Three Rehabilitation, you will use the equipment that you are already familiar with such as the torture rack, the tormentor, etc. Only now you can change up your routine do things in different sequence, and length of time on each piece of equipment, compared to what you did before.

You will probably get to use new equipment that you may not have been able to use in Phase Two, and you probably will not have to wear "The Box." No doubt, you will be weighed from time to time. In my program, it was (is) once a month. We also have an EKG done once a month and get a strip to take with us. (no guys, not that kind) an EKG strip.

You may wear a strap and a pulse monitor that will monitor your pulse while you are exercising. You will also have your blood pressure (BP) taken when you arrive, in the middle of your workout, and before you leave. You will still do your warm ups and cool downs. Sorry, I tried to talk them out of it. Depending on your target heart rate you will be given a pulse rate to shoot for while you work to strengthen your heart and body.

Your cardiologist will suggest your target heart rate. This may require a stress test first, to help determine what your target pulse rate will be.

You will have more flexibility in the hours that you choose to go to cardio rehabilitation, and in the length of time that you exercise. You will meet new friends while still seeing some of your Phase Two friends. You will be monitored at all times with the same degree of skill and dedication that you experienced in Phase Two, probably by the same staff that you have come to know and love.

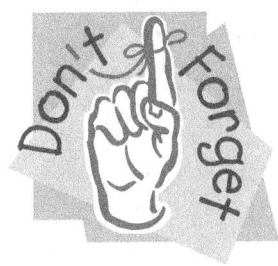

Remember..

Phase One was what led up to your event and the event itself; treatments made and care given.

Phase Two was rehabilitation to help you get better, stronger and back to doing the things you love to do, learning what may have contributed to your health issues and ways to combat a recurrence by doing such things as, exercise, developing better eating habits, gaining knowledge about your cholesterol levels, diabetes, managing stress, taking proper medications, the importance of routine doctor visits and follow-ups. Phase Two rehab also gives you the knowledge to understand what has happened to you and what to look for. It teaches you to pay attention to how you feel at rest, during exercise and after a workout. It gives you information that will help you around the clock in listening to what your body is telling you in order to lessen the chance of a recurrence and prompt you to seek medical advice immediately should you have any issues or questions.

Phase Three is ongoing continued heart and body rehabilitation to enable you to be as healthy as you can be! It is an ongoing commitment by your health care providers to give you all the tools, information, guidance, patience, and encouragement that you need to continue your journey to wellness.

COMMIT TO CARDIAC PHASE THREE

You and only you can make the commitment to continue on with your journey. You have come a long way and it makes perfect sense to continue on to better health. It takes hard work on your part but the benefits are GREAT. You have been through a traumatic and difficult time and anything that you can do NOW to benefit yourself, your loved ones, and more importantly, your HEART is a huge plus for you and those you love. Please, please do so. Ask your cardio team about on-going Phase Three Rehabilitation today. You will be so glad that you did and your heart will thank you.

CARDIAC DISEASE

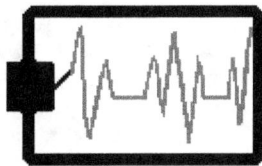

I have heard it said that one in three adults has some form of cardiovascular disease or heart related issues. Many people have high blood pressure that goes untreated! What about high cholesterol? Look, I can go on and on, but heart disease and heart related problems know no boundaries or age group. Heart disease affects people of all races, ages, sizes, shapes, and sex. But a lot of what you can do NOW, may narrow your chance of problems later and increase your overall quality of life.

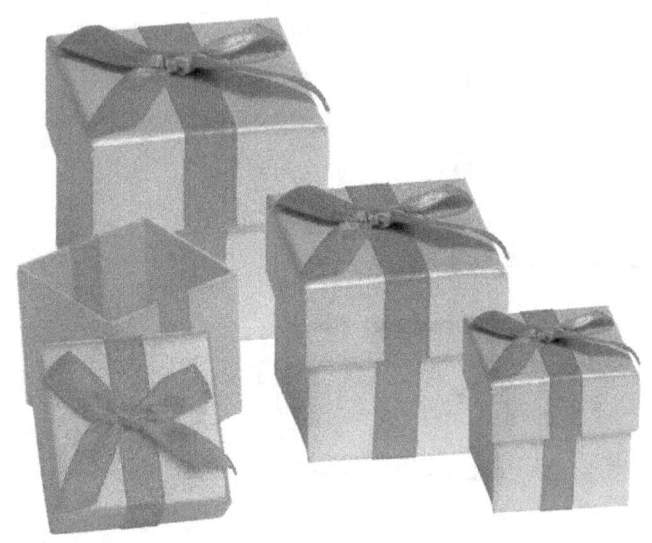

GIVE YOURSELF A GIFT:
I have heard these things over and over and so have you. But we need to pay attention, because they make a difference.

- Eat right.
- Watch your weight.
- Relax more.
- Have regular doctor visits.
- EXERCISE for a period of at least 30-45 minutes at least three times a week. Walking is a great exercise.

- Be careful with the amount of alcohol and caffeine that you consume.
- Drink plenty of water.
- Don't Smoke.
- Get at least 8 hrs of sleep a night.
- Make time for you.

All the things I have just listed plus some I probably neglected to mention are more important now than ever before. Although not always so easy to do but, by taking the advice we have heard over and over you will be on the way to a healthier you and you will be so glad that you did.

DON'T HESITATE TO GET HELP

Always, I repeat, always seek medical treatment should you have any symptoms of a heart related problem or for that matter any medical emergency! CALL 911. Seek help immediately. Do not wait! Seconds count and can mean the difference between life and death. Do not hesitate ever to make the call. If you have a health problem make yourself as knowledgeable as you possibly can about your condition.

BE A PROFESSOR OF YOUR OWN HEALTH

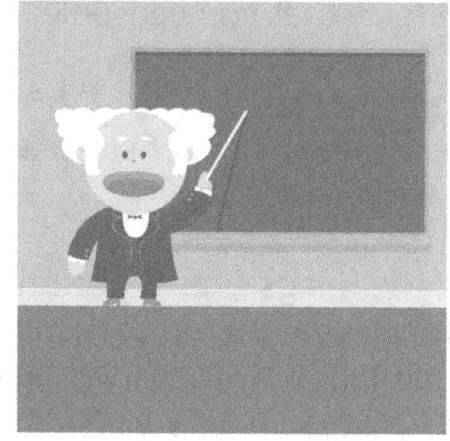

I don't care what it is; it doesn't matter how long you have had it or what has been done regarding treatment. Strive to become a professor of your health issues! Know as much as you can about what you have, what's being done, and what you can do to help prevent it from happening again, but most importantly: LEARN WHAT YOU CAN DO TO ENHANCE AND INCREASE THE QUALITY OF YOUR LIFE AND HEALTHY WELL-BEING. DO IT FOR YOU!!!! YOU DESERVE IT my friends you deserve it.

CHECK WITH YOUR DOCTORS FIRST

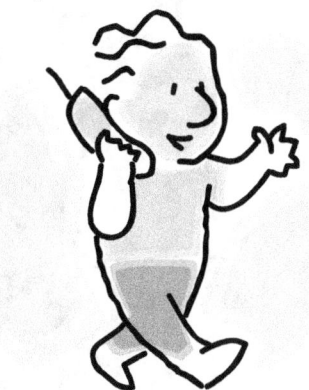

Some of you may not sign on to a monitored environment to continue your well-being trip. You may decide to do it on your own, you may decide to go to a gym instead, or you may decide to wait a bit before attempting any more exercise or additional services. Whatever your choice, please follow the guidelines and advice of your doctor and health care providers before starting any routine on your own. Please always seek expert advice from a health care professional!

WE'RE IN THIS TOGETHER

I am just a patient like you trying to get better. Like you, I seek advice as well. And I believe that by following the advice of our caregivers, 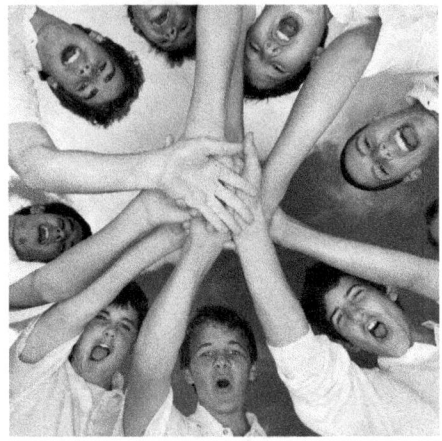 doctors, and with all the information that is available to us about our conditions, that together we can achieve many wonderful things. We're in this together.

THE GIFT OF A NEW DAY

Take just a small moment every day to look around you and look at all that God has done for you. See the leaves gently blowing

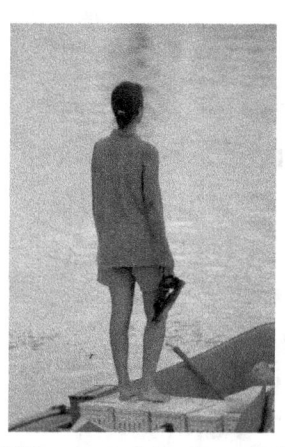 in the trees. Watch the gentle snow glisten through the sun. Breathe in the wonderful smell of fresh turned earth in spring. See a flower wake up so you can smell it. Watch a fawn follow its mother across a meadow full of all

different kinds of flowers. See the joy on a child's face and the wonder in his eyes as he listens to a story or does something for the very first time. Watch a bird in flight. Count the different shapes of clouds. Smell and taste a babbling mountain stream. Take a walk down a dusty old road. Get a call from an old friend. Tell someone, "Good job." Go fishing and don't worry if you don't catch anything.

HAPPY MOMENTS..

There are so many happy moments, thoughts, memories, and wonderful things to see, hear, touch and do every day that can give you a wonderful feeling. Listen to your heart!

Reach up your hand. Look to the sky and say, "Thank you, Lord." Sometimes, we just seem to get too busy with everyday life to see the wonders of each day. So let the door open to the lost child within you. Wonder about life and enjoy the many beautiful things around you that may just have slipped your mind. Give thanks that you have been given another day. It is a gift from God.

ARE YOU TREADING ON THIN ICE?

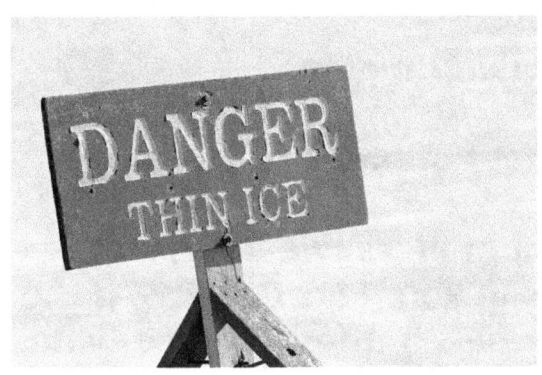

PAY ATTENTION TO THESE HEART DISEASE SYMPTOMS

Remember, heart disease symptoms will vary depending on what type of heart disease you have.

Cardiovascular disease is caused by narrowed, blocked or stiffened blood vessels that prevent your heart, brain or other parts of your body from receiving enough blood.

Cardiovascular disease symptoms can include:

♥ Chest pain (angina)

♥ Shortness of breath

♥ Pain, numbness, weakness or coldness in your legs or arms, if the blood vessels in those parts of your body are narrowed.

By not having regular doctor visits, you might not be diagnosed with cardio vascular disease until your condition worsens to the point that you have a heart attack, angina, stroke, or heart failure. So schedule that check-up today.

It's important to watch for cardiovascular symptoms and discuss any concerns with your doctor. Cardiovascular disease can sometimes be found early with regular visits to your doctor. As it is for any disease, the sooner it is found, the better your chance for survival.

DON'T WAIT

If you are experiencing cardiac symptoms, seek help immediately. In an emergency, call 911. It is better to be safe than sorry.

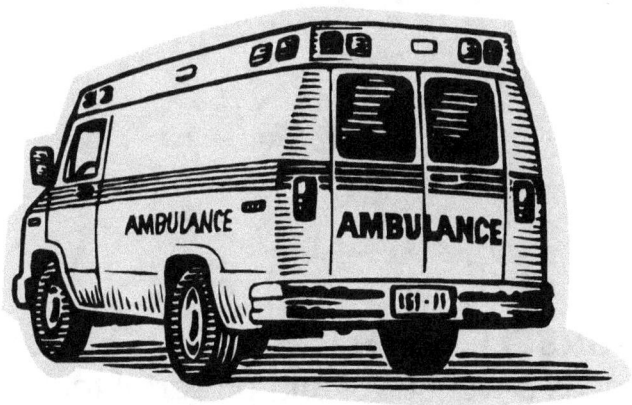

ARM YOURSELF WITH KNOWLEDGE

Knowledge is a wonderful and powerful tool in your journey to wellness. The more you know and understand, the better prepared you are to make a wise decision. In my own quest, I read books and did a fair amount of web surfing. I asked many questions and talked to others like myself who have had heart related issues.

I do not endorse any of the sites I will list or places I have been, however they have been extremely useful to me and I am very grateful for that. All works and thoughts in this book are based on my own experiences, I am not a doctor nor do I pretend to be. I am a heart patient like yourself, sharing my trials and tribulations, my ups and downs, my joys and sorrows, my triumphs and defeats, my laughter and my tears.

A GREAT TIME TO LIVE

We live in a great time. No matter where you live quality health care is just around the corner with great doctors, nurses , and a team of professionals, ready and willing to serve you. Modern medicine has made great strides and the new advancements and quality of care continues to grow every day. Your providers can refer you to a world of specialized professionals, each unique in their own field of expertise.

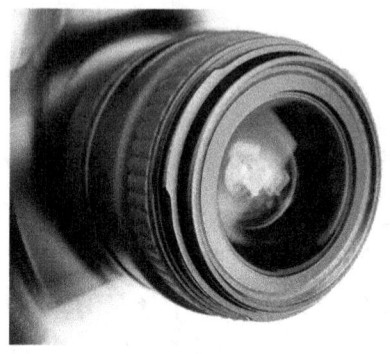

FOCUS ON GETTING WELL

You can and will be encouraged to get other specialist involved in your case if need be. I would politely ask you to not worry about costs and focus your attention instead on getting well and leave the insurance and other costs involved to one of the many agencies that can guide you. Yes, there are many agencies that will guide you in getting the help that you need. You sometimes need to keep pushing and looking.

Your health care providers can also direct you to resources that may be available to you. Always put your health first and the rest will get sorted out later. You will have to make choices some hard but you are the patient and it is your health we are talking about. I am not trying to scare you, although it may not be a bad idea if it helps you stay healthy. Use the many wonderful tools around you everyday to help you achieve wellness.

WEBSITES

The following is a short list of websites that helped me to learn more about my condition and treatment options. There are many more out there. Always seek your doctor's advice and ask questions about your condition. Do a little research on your own but always consult with your doctor before making decisions. Make informed choices with your healthcare providers and share your thoughts and questions with them.

POSSIBLE RESOURCES TO CHECK OUT

www. mayoclinic.com
www. clevelandclinic.org
www. medicine net.com
www.healthdesk.com
www.heart.org:
The American Heart Association

I gratefully acknowledge the sites listed above and although THIS IS NOT AN ENDORSEMENT, THEY WERE VERY HELPFUL TO ME. You can also use the internet to search for your own local resources.

OTHER RESOURCES

Also check your local library. Larger cities often have medical libraries and medical universities and all are a wealth of knowledge. But none as important as your trained, skilled team of professionals, and you.

A TEAM OF CARING PROFESSIONALS
Think of everyone who helped you during your cardiac crisis.
From the professionals at the 911 Center..

To the transport provided by local volunteer

and/or paid emergency services..

To the Medical Technicians..

To the Advanced Life Support Team...

To the Emergency Room staff...

To the doctors, nurses and support staff ..

To the staff of the Recovery room..

To the staff of the Intensive care unit..

To the therapists, nutritionists..

To the housekeeping, aides, chaplains, etc.

Everyone you met along the way as quiet or hectic as things may have become had your best interest at heart and they did and will continue to do, all that they can, to assure a quality outcome.

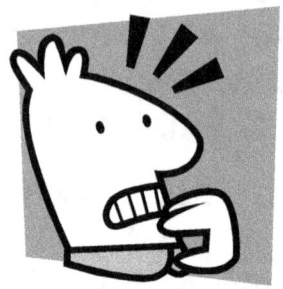

DON'T BE AFRAID TO SPEAK UP!
Sure we have all heard stories of procedures that didn't go as planned or that the outcome was not what was expected. Sometimes even the best surgeons, offering the best quality of care are no match for advanced disease or multiple trauma and unforeseen circumstances that happen during surgery or treatment. Sometimes what is broken, can't be fixed.

But remember, you have a say and you need to speak up when you feel your care or the care of a loved one is in question. Sometimes things are not what they seem and other times they may be exactly as they seem. You have a voice. Make it heard. When in doubt, speak up.

SPEAK UP: IT'S YOUR RIGHT

You have a right to speak up. Ask questions and if you think that something is wrong, keep on it. People know themselves better than 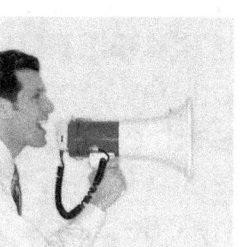 the doctor, so again, make your thoughts known.

FEEDBACK IS IMPORTANT

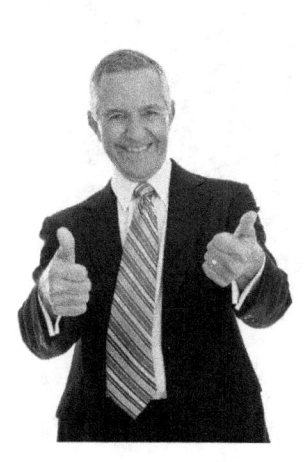 Health Care Facilities strive to deliver the very best in care. They want to know your concerns. They want to improve on the quality of care you receive and they want your honest feedback to constantly strive to be the best at what they do, big or small. We need and expect the highest level of quality care that is possible, but we also must take care of ourselves at the same time.

ULTIMATELY IT'S YOUR RESPONSIBILTY

You have the responsibility to become healthier and you should always follow your Health Care Provider's advice. If you have any questions, get a second opinion. But with all the wonderful advances in medicine, you are ultimately the one who must make the healthy choice or not.

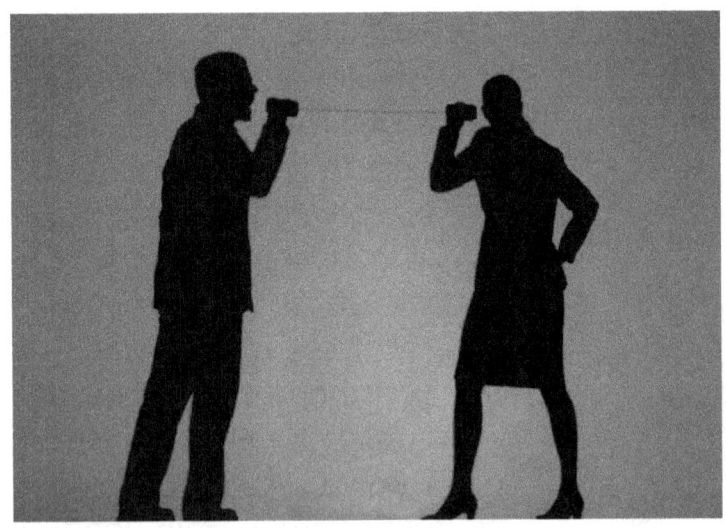

YES, I'M REPEATING MYSELF...

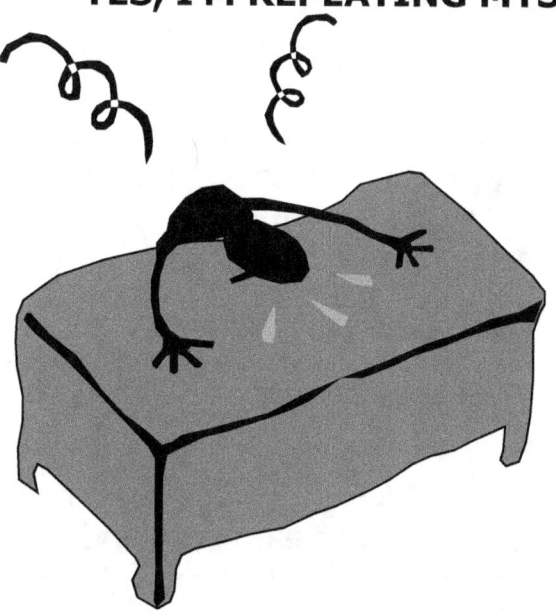

You will notice that at times, I have repeated myself throughout this book.   I did this only to ensure that you understand the points that I am trying to make. And because I know that it will bug some of you. (Ha ha!!) Remember, YOU are the important one when it comes to your care and treatment. It is about YOU! The more you know and listen and work on getting well, the better you will be.

LOOKING TOWARD A BRIGHTER TOMORROW

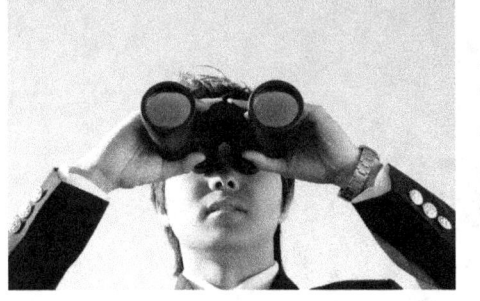

It's really amazing how many advances that there have been in medicine in the past few years. Moreover, new discoveries are being made each and every day. Researchers are uncovering new information that in turn, leads to new treatments and therapies. In the field of cardiac care alone, procedures such as valve replacement, bypass surgery, and even heart transplants, are fairly common. A generation ago, who would have dreamed that these treatments would have even been possible? So what I'm saying is no matter what your condition is, hold on to hope. Perhaps, a treatment for your disease is on the horizon.

GIVE THE GIFT OF LIFE

Have you thought about giving the gift of life through an organ donation program? Your physician can provide you with the information and paperwork that needs to be completed to get the ball rolling.

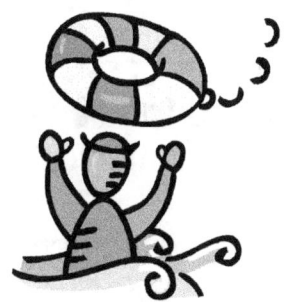

DISCLAIMER:

The information provided in this book should not be used during any medical emergency or for the diagnosis or treatment of any medical condition.

A licensed medical professional should always be consulted for diagnosis and treatment of any and all medical conditions.

Call 911 for all medical emergencies.

Links to other sites are provided for information only -- they do not constitute endorsements of those other sites.

Any similarities between the author of this book and any other person living or dead is purely coincidental and they have my deepest sympathy.

Thank you and be well!

Steve Wickman

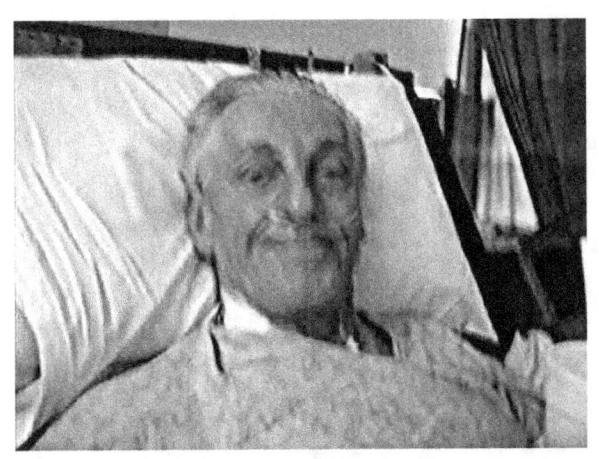

HERE I AM ABOUT 36 HOURS AFTER SURGERY

(I LOOKED AND FELT LIKE CRAP!)

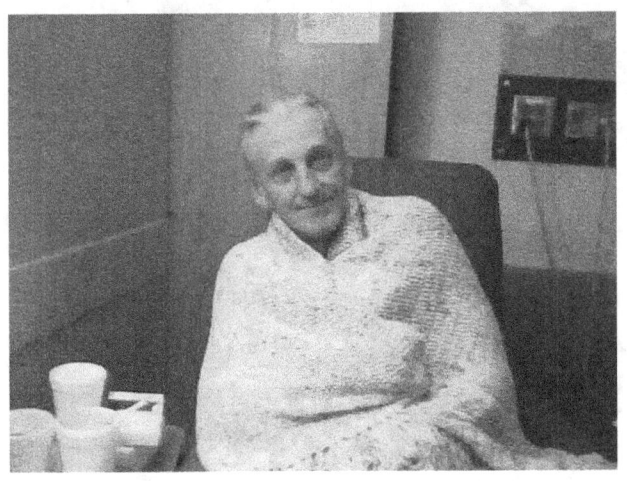

WRAPPED IN MY PRAYER SHAWL

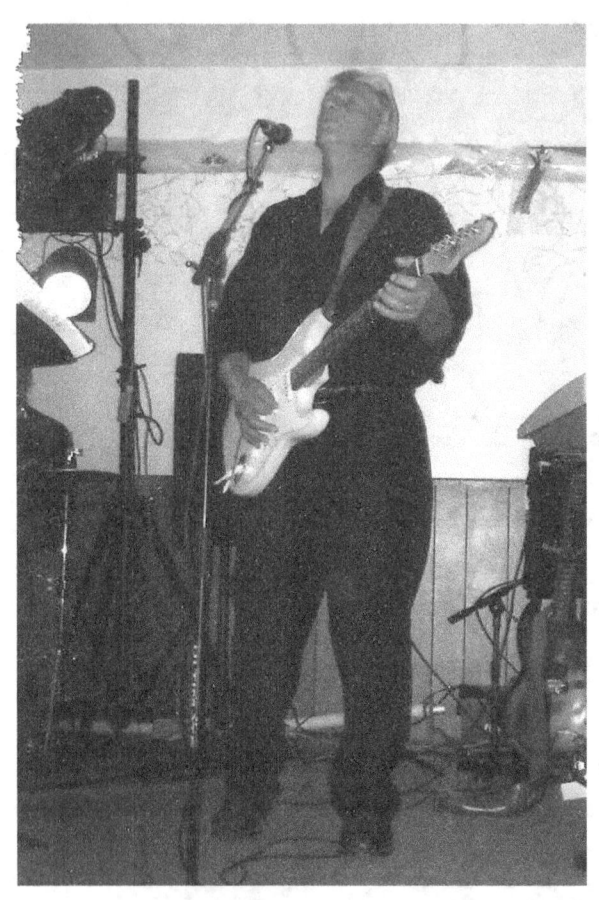

**SINGING AGAIN!!
THANK YOU TO EVERYONE WHO
HELPED ME ON MY JOURNEY TO
WELLNESS.**

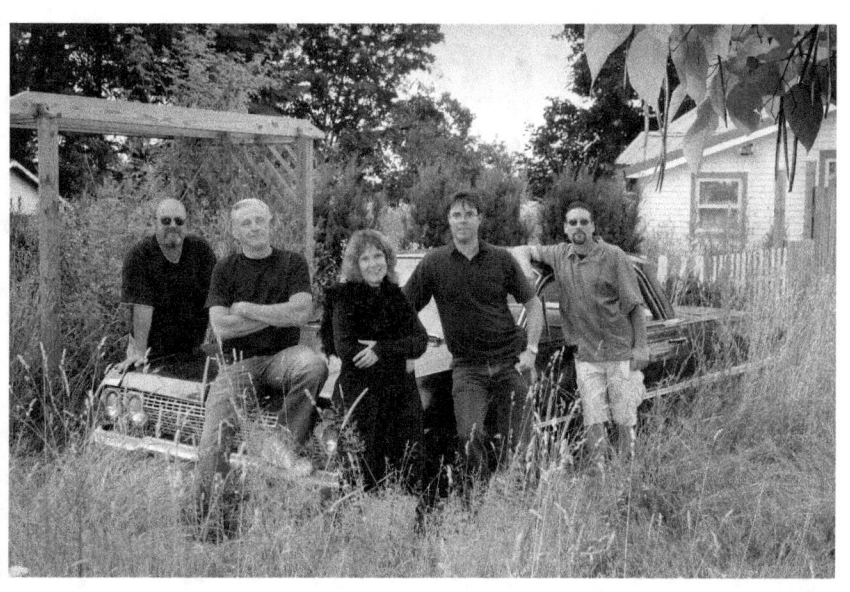

MAKING MUSIC AGAIN WITH
SOME OF MY FRIENDS
LEFT TO RIGHT: PETE, ME, CYNTHIA, JAY AND FRED

THANKS FOR
RIDING ALONG WITH ME
IN MY JOURNEY TO WELLNESS.
BEST WISHES TO YOU!
-Steve

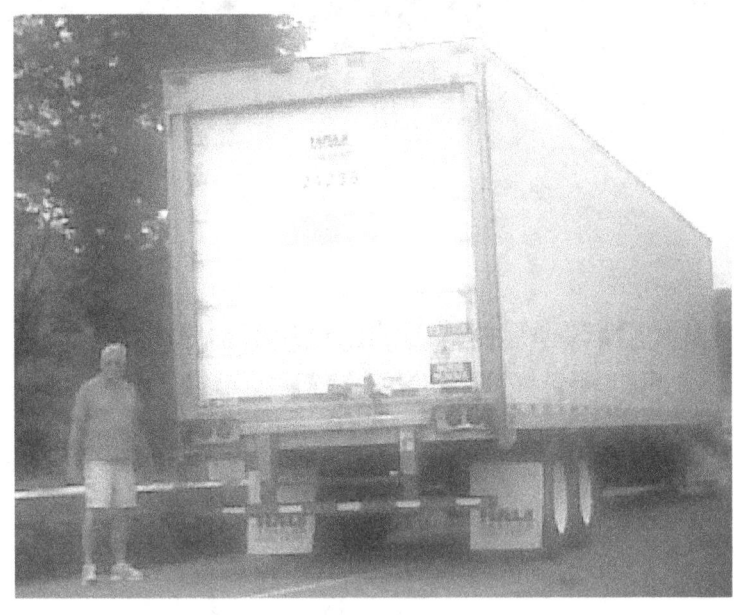

Back on the Road Again!

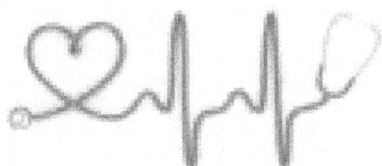

A PORTION OF THE PROCEEDS OF THIS
BOOK WILL BE DONATED TO
THE **"STEVE WICKMAN SPEAK FROM
THE HEART FUND."** THE FUND
PROVIDES A RESOURCE TO THOSE WHO
NEED FINANCIAL ASSISTANCE TO PAY FOR
CARDIAC REHABILITAION AND/OR SPEECH
REHABILITATION SERVICES. THE FUND IS
SET UP THROUGH THE ROCHESTER
GENERAL FOUNDATION.

WWW.GIVERGH.ORG
SELECT PERSONAL FUNDRAISING
SELECT: STEPHEN K. WICKMAN, SR.
SPEAK FROM THE HEART

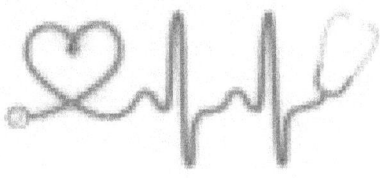

RECORD YOUR IMPORTANT
MEDICAL INFORMATION
ON THE FOLLOWING PAGES

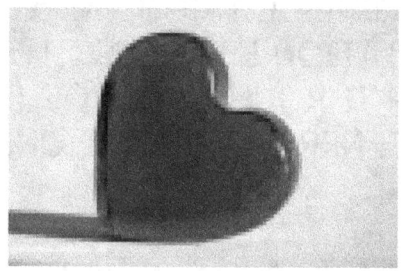

Charting Your Blood Pressure and Pulse

Date	B/P am	Pulse am	B/P pm	Pulse pm	comments

Charting Your Blood Pressure and Pulse

Date	B/P am	Pulse am	B/P pm	Pulse pm	comments

My Medication List
Bring this list to every doctor's appointment!!
Ask Your Doctor to Review what you are taking!

Medication:_____
Strength_____
What is this medicine for?_____
Dosage(how often do you take this medicine?
_____
Prescribed by_____
Date Prescribed_____
Remarks:_____

Medication:_____
Strength_____
What is this medicine for?_____
Dosage(how often do you take this medicine?
_____
Prescribed by_____
Date Prescribed_____
Remarks:_____

Medication:_____
Strength_____
What is this medicine for?_____
Dosage(how often do you take this medicine?
_____
Prescribed by_____
Remarks:_____

YOUR ALLERGIES: TELL YOUR DRS & PHARMACIST

My Medication List
Bring this list to every doctor's appointment!!
Ask Your Doctor to Review what you are taking

Medication:_____

Strength_____

What is this medicine for?_____

Dosage(how often do you take this medicine?

_____

Prescribed by_____

Date Prescribed_____

Remarks:_____

Medication:_____

Strength_____

What is this medicine for?_____

Dosage(how often do you take this medicine?

_____

Prescribed by_____

Date Prescribed_____

Remarks:_____

Medication:_____

Strength_____

What is this medicine for?_____

Dosage(how often do you take this medicine?

_____

Prescribed by_____

Remarks:_____

186

My Medication List
Bring this list to every doctor's appointment!!
Ask Your Doctor to Review what you are taking

Medication:_____
Strength_____
What is this medicine for?_____
Dosage(how often do you take this medicine?
_____
Prescribed by_____
Date Prescribed_____
Remarks:_____

Medication:_____
Strength_____
What is this medicine for?_____
Dosage(how often do you take this medicine?
_____
Prescribed by_____
Date Prescribed_____
Remarks:_____

Medication:_____
Strength_____
What is this medicine for?_____
Dosage(how often do you take this medicine?
_____
Prescribed by_____
Remarks:_____

My Medication List
Bring this list to every doctor's appointment!!
Ask Your Doctor to Review what you are taking

Medication:_____

Strength_____

What is this medicine for?_____

Dosage(how often do you take this medicine?

_____

Prescribed by_____

Date Prescribed_____

Remarks:_____

_____

Medication:_____

Strength_____

What is this medicine for?_____

Dosage(how often do you take this medicine?

_____

Prescribed by_____

Date Prescribed_____

Remarks:_____

Medication:_____

Strength_____

What is this medicine for?_____

Dosage(how often do you take this medicine?

_____

Prescribed by_____

Remarks:_____

_____

MY DAILY MEDICINE REMINDER

CHECK ✓ AFTER YOU TAKE YOUR MEDS!!

DATE	MORNING MEDS?	AFTERNOON MEDS?	EVENING MEDS?	OTHER

MY DAILY MEDICINE REMINDER

CHECK ✔ AFTER YOU TAKE YOUR MEDS!!

DATE	MORNING MEDS?	AFTERNOON MEDS?	EVENING MEDS?	OTHER

Important Phone Numbers

Emergencies- CALL 911

*Your Primary Care Physician_____

Phone Number_____

* Your Cardiologist_____

Phone Number_____

* Your Pharmacy_____

Phone Number_____

Your Hospital_____

Phone Number_____

Your Emergency Contact Information:

_____   _____
Name (relationship)   Phone numbers

_____   _____
Name (relationship)   Phone numbers

_____   _____
Name (relationship)   Phone numbers

Other Numbers

_____   _____
Contact   Phone Number

_____   _____
Contact   Phone Number

Acknowledgements & Sources

Borg, GA. "Psychophysical Bases of Perceived Exertion." Medicine and Sports Exercise 1982; 14:377-381

Photo Credits: Selected photos purchased from IStockphoto.com. Also used Microsoft Office media images and clip art: used with permission from Microsoft.

For additional information on how you can help those in need of financial assistance for rehabilitation services, through the **Steve Wickman Speak From the Heart Fund**, through the Rochester General Foundation, please visit:

http://www.givergh.org

♥ Remember the best source of health information is from your own primary health care providers.

NOTES

NOTES

NOTES

NOTES

www.ingramcontent.com/pod-product-compliance
Lightning Source LLC
Chambersburg PA
CBHW062158280526
45788CB00001B/356